The Savvy Resident's Guide:
Everything You Wanted to Know About Your Nursing Home Stay But Were Afraid to Ask

The Savvy Resident's Guide:
Everything You Wanted to Know About Your Nursing Home Stay But Were Afraid to Ask

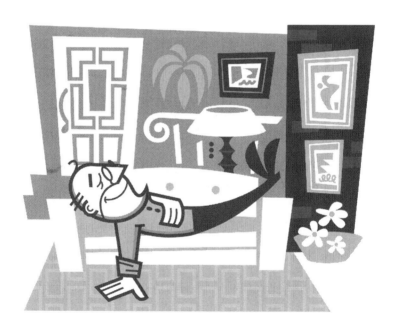

Eleanor Feldman Barbera, PhD

Visit Dr. El at
MyBetterNursingHome.com

The Savvy Resident's Guide:
Everything You Wanted to Know
About Your Nursing Home Stay
But Were Afraid to Ask

ISBN: 978-0-9854054-0-3
© 2012 Psychology Insights Press/
Eleanor Feldman Barbera

Cover and interior design:
Gretchen Mergenthaler/ThingsIHaveDesigned.com

Cover illustration: www.peterbajohr.com
(also used in the interior)

Author photograph: BluFace Photography

This book is dedicated to my peeps
—past, present, and future.
Thank you for sharing your lives with me.

Contents

CONTENTS

Sidebars

Foreword

For Residents:

For over fifteen years as a psychologist in long-term care, I've helped residents negotiate the nursing home and create meaning and purpose out of their nursing home stays. In this guidebook, I address common concerns of residents like you. You'll discover important information it could otherwise take months to learn and find ways to resolve and/or cope with problems that arise. Join me, and several "residents" created from the voices of real people I've known while working in long-term care facilities, as we tour the nursing home.

If you're new to long-term care, I recommend beginning with the "Introduction" and "Quick Start" chapters, and then reading on as you're ready. If you've been in a nursing home for a while, you'll find the book will confirm what you've experienced (you're not alone!), increase your understanding of how things work and why, and provide coping skills you might not have tried. If you think your family members might benefit from the book, consider reading or sharing it with them. My goal in writing this book is for your time in a nursing home to be one of growth and contentment. I hope The Savvy Resident's Guide helps you along the way.

For Family Members:

Entering a nursing home can be over-whelming and confusing for everyone involved. Although written for residents, this book also provides answers to many of your own questions, as well as strategies to assist your loved one during their nursing home stay. Some residents will appreciate being given this guidebook as a gift and will read it on their own. Others will need your help to find the information they need and your encouragement to use the sugges-tions I've given. Just like in my bedside psychotherapy sessions, most residents find it very helpful to know that others have been in the same situations and felt the same ways they have. Reading the stories of my composite residents will be for your loved one like finding knowledgeable friends willing to share their experiences.

For Staff:

Do you remember your first days in long-term care with new people, medical equipment, and jargon? Now imagine experiencing those days without training and when you're not feeling well. The Savvy Resident's Guide is a tool for residents (and their families) to bring order to those chaotic early days and to make sense of the nursing home. The book functions as a readily available team member, fielding questions and saving time so you can provide care in other ways. It offers information and strategies so that readers can become calm, knowledgeable, and proactive members of the treatment team.

The Savvy Resident's Guide makes an ideal addition to the nursing home's "Welcome Package." The topics addressed in *The Savvy Guide* can be used for group discussions with residents and families in forums such as resident and family council meetings or resident education program.

For All:

One of the things I like most about my work as a nursing home psychologist is that I literally learn something new every day. This book is based on my experiences working with residents in various nursing homes in New York City, my extensive reading in the field, and my discussions with others living and working in nursing homes in numerous locations. If something I've written is unclear, or different where you are, please let me know. If there are areas I've missed (and I'm sure there are), please write, and I'll try to add them to the next edition.

By working together, I know we can make nursing homes better.

All the best on your journey,
Dr. El
Eleanor Feldman Barbera, PhD

My Better Nursing Home
http://mybetternursinghome.com
drel@mybetternursinghome.com

Acknowledgements

With thanks to Marc Agronin, Peter Bajohr, Taylor Barton, Sandy Beadle, Martine Bellen, Robin Bonifas, Dale Carter, Jill Cohen, Catherine Crowley, Bill Curran, Rema Famorca, Beth Levy Feigenblatt, Lisa Gallagher, Fred Gleeck, Jane Gross, Maggie Hadleigh-West, Mark Kissinger, Kevin Kolus, Frank La Mendola, Kathleen Mears, Gretchen Mergenthaler, Victoria Moran, Bill O'Hanlon, Avish Parashar, Jamie Pesavento, Oliver Sacks, Sue Samek, David Solie, Nilesh Soni, Cassis Staudt, Wendy Wu, my writers group buddies over the years, and others who contributed their ideas and support along the way. With special thanks to my family.

The Savvy Resident's Guide: Everything You Wanted to Know About Your Nursing Home Stay But Were Afraid to Ask

Great Idea!

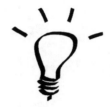

Throughout this book I have put this bright light to indicate that there is a **great idea** in the text next to it.

Dr. El

Introduction:
Welcome to the Nursing Home

"Well, I've finally reached the end of the road." John sighed, looking around the small area now known as home.

I'd closed the privacy curtain that separates his bed from his roommate's side of the room during our psychotherapy session, though it didn't offer much privacy. Below a corkboard containing the photocopied recreation calendar was a brown dresser, its smooth top reflecting the fluorescent glow of the light over his bed. Floral curtains matched the border on the wallpaper and highlighted the color of the bedspread. The room contained nothing that showed John had a life prior to admission to the nursing home three days ago.

I followed his gaze around the room. "John, this may feel like the end of the road, but I've been working in nursing homes for a long time and I can tell you that this is just the beginning of a new part of the journey."

Most people reading this guidebook probably wish they weren't in a nursing home and would prefer not to be welcomed to this strange new world. Life being what it is, we often find ourselves in unexpected circumstances. As you've no doubt learned along the way, it's our approach to situations that makes the biggest difference in the experience. The skills that have helped you through past challenges will help you here too.

Whether your stay is short or long, you are here, and you've been given this day. This guidebook will make the nursing home world more comfortable and familiar and give you tools for making the most of your time here.

You'll notice that I refer to the nursing home as a "world." That's how I see it. The floor you're on is your neighborhood, and your roommate is your next-door neighbor. The staff members are coworkers in the job of getting you ready to face each day. You may be retired, but there is work to be done!

Chapter 1

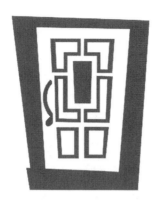

Quick Start Guide:
What to Expect upon Your Arrival

It's totally normal to feel overwhelmed when you first arrive at the nursing home.

"Who the hell are you?" Vivian asked me before I even had a chance to knock on her open door.

"I'm the psychologist."

"Well, you're the fifth person coming by in an hour, and I can't keep track any more. I suppose you want to ask me the same questions as everyone else."

"Probably," I admitted. "But I'll try to be nice about it."

Initial Assessments

When you first get to the nursing home, the staff members will want to get to know you. You can expect representatives of various departments to visit and ask you lots of personal questions, many of which will be the same. As frustrating as that can be, the goal is to provide you with the best service possible. Try to answer the questions as accurately as you can because information tends to get repeated once it's written in the chart. If you're feeling tired or not up for questions, it's okay to ask the staff person to come back later or to have someone in your family answer questions for you.

Rehabilitation

When you first arrive at the nursing home, you'll be evaluated by the rehabilitation department and will very likely be referred for some type of exercise to improve your physical condition. While some residents are extremely motivated to begin this type of treatment, many are not. They don't feel like going to physical therapy, doubt it will

2

help them, and they just want to stay in bed and sleep. Is that you? If I just described your thoughts, please be sure to read this section and chapter 5: "What Rehabilitation Can Do for You."

Rehab is the most important thing you can do for yourself when you enter the nursing home. So many people have rolled in and walked out! It can happen for you! Don't let your depression trick you into believing it isn't worth the effort. Even if rehab doesn't get you on your feet again, it can make a huge difference in your quality of life and make you more independent.

Most insurance companies and Medicare and Medicaid pay for a brief period of rehabilitation while you're making progress, and then you're no longer eligible to be covered for treatment unless there's a change in your condition. It's vital to make the most of this window of opportunity. So what can you do when you don't much feel like trying?

Staffing: Who's Who

So many uniforms! Your main staff people when you arrive at the nursing home will include:

Certified Nursing Assistants
(CNAs or Aides, sometimes referred to as Personal Care Assistants). Aides assist with bathing, dressing, feeding, and other "activities of daily living."

Nurses

The Medication Nurse gives out medication.

The Charge Nurse talks with your medical doctor, keeps track of appointments, and is generally "in charge" of the flow of the unit.

The Nursing Supervisor is responsible for the residents living on several floors and can assist with issues that have not been resolved by the nurses and aides on your unit.

Rehabilitation Staff

    The Physical Therapist exercises your lower body.

    The Occupational Therapist exercises your upper body.

The Social Worker helps you settle in, stays in contact with your family, and plans your discharge.

The Recreation Therapist guides you to find activities in the nursing home that suits your interests.

The Dietitian makes sure you have meals and snacks that fit your diet and preferences.

Your Medical Doctor orders every medication and service you receive at the nursing home. Though you might not see the doctor as often as you'd expect, the nurses keep the doctor closely informed about your condition.

Tell yourself "it's now or never" and muster up the strength and courage to do your best.

Stick with the winners by observing the people in therapy with determination and a positive attitude. Avoid those who are just going through the motions. Attitude is contagious.

Read the rehabilitation chapter (chapter 5) for more tips.

The Adjustment Period

Entering a nursing home is distressing for most people. **Be gentle with yourself, and give yourself time.** Utilize the following supports:

Spiritual: Every nursing home has religious services of many different religions. Attending them can be like taking a survey course in world religion.

"My mother always told me, 'It doesn't matter how you pray,' so I go to

all the services," 90-year-old Clarice said matter-of-factly.

Friends and Family: Encourage your friends and family to visit. Ask someone to call people you know to give them your contact information.

> *"I can't do that!" Miguel protested.*
> *"Then I'll do it for you. Who do you know who wouldn't mind making a few phone calls?"*
> *He thought a moment, and I could see his discomfort with relying on others battling it out with his need for contact. Finally, he said, "Well, my cousin Maria knows who to reach in my family, and if you call Herbie, he'll let the guys from the bar know what happened to me."*
> *"Great." A few minutes later I'd mobilized a chain of phone calls and visitors that lasted the length of Miguel's nursing home stay.*

Staff Members: The staff of every department is there to ensure you're as comfortable as possible. If you're feeling depressed or anxious, ask to talk with the social worker. She can also refer you to the psychologist, if needed.

Other Residents: Talking to others in your situation can be a great way to add some humor and perspective.

"Are you able to meet now?" I asked Mary when I ran into her in the hallway a few weeks after her admission.

"Oh dear. I promised I'd meet a lady at quilting class."

"No worries, Mary. I'll catch you later, after the class is over."

She appeared relieved. "I appreciate your help, don't get me wrong," she told me, "but this lady and I are both from down south and, well, she just knows what it's like..."

"I understand. Friends are the best way to make it here, Mary. Enjoy."

Learn How to Respond to Residents with Dementia

Two main symptoms of dementia are:

- Rummaging through people's things
- Wandering

Due to their illness, residents with dementia occasionally enter the wrong room and look in the drawers, which can be distressing and sometimes frightening. To reduce your worry about your belongings, put your important items in a locked drawer. If a resident with dementia has wandered into your room, rather than ask them to leave, tell them they're needed down the hall or that the nurse wants to see them. Just like most of us, people with dementia are more likely to comply with a positive request and to get irritated by a demand. If it's a repeated problem, you can ask the nurse or social worker to put up a "stop sign," which is a removable banner that runs across your doorway, acting as a deterrent to entering the room.

Residents with dementia are often frightened because the world has become unfamiliar. Being kind to them can work wonders.

Chapter 2

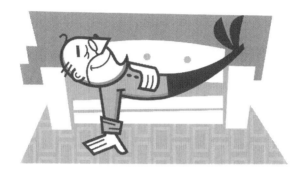

Coming Out of Retirement:
Working with the Staff

Different Shifts

One of the most important aspects of nursing home life is the flow of the workday. Most nursing homes have three shifts of nurses and aides that provide you with direct care. Usually the shifts run from:

7 a.m. to 3 p.m.
3 p.m. to 11 p.m.
11 p.m. to 7 a.m.

Some homes have different staff on the weekends.

There will be many people caring for you during your stay, including staff that will cover when your regular aide or nurse is on vacation or taking a day off. The good news about having so many different people around to help is that you're very likely to find several folks with whom you have a good personality match. With some staff members you'll have a strictly business relationship and others can become almost like family.

"Precious is on tonight," Clarice said. "That's her name, but it really is true. She treats me like her own mother. She comes in at 7 and leaves at 3. I always know her schedule."

Another lady once said, "Some of the workers are like angels sent from above. Others are from hell." It's a sentiment I've heard echoed over the years. Find your angels.

Chain of Command

Certified Nursing Assistant (CNA)
|
Medication Nurse
|
Charge Nurse
|
Nursing Supervisor
|
Director of Nursing

There can be a confusing sea of uniforms (and acronyms) in a nursing home. The Certified Nursing Assistants (CNAs) are those responsible for your basic care, like washing, dressing, and toileting. The CNAs are supervised by the nurses on the floor. Often there will be one nurse who gives out medication (the Medication Nurse), and one nurse who is in charge of other aspects of care (the Charge Nurse).

The nurses have Nursing Supervisors who oversee their work. Each Nursing Supervisor is in charge of several floors or units. The Nursing Department has a Director of Nursing, and often an Assistant Director of Nursing, who is guiding them.

Most of the time, you'll be working with your aides and the nurses on the floor, but be assured that if you have an issue that you're unable to work out with them, there is always someone you can turn to for help.

Busy Times

Nursing homes are busy places, and there are certain times of the day when your aide is less likely to be available. Though it's not always possible, if you are able to **plan your needs around the busy times,** you'll find yourself getting care more quickly and with fewer frustrating waits.

The aides and nurses are busiest during mealtimes and especially at the change of shift. For example, if the change of shift in your nursing home is at 3 p.m., it's going be most difficult to get care between 2:30 p.m. and 3:30 p.m. because the day aides are finishing up their work to go home and the evening aides are just settling in. If you can, ask for what you need well before or after mealtimes and the change of shift window. The aides have many residents to take care of, so pretend you're at a large party with only one bathroom, and get on line early!

"I tried your party thing and it worked," John told me the week after we'd discussed his frustration with the long waits for help. "Yep, I knew I was going to need care before the first shift left, so I pushed my call bell with plenty of time for them to answer it. Then I just sat and read the paper."

"So no aggravation and high blood pressure this time?"

"I still hate having to ask for help, but it was a lot better. And I didn't have to apologize for my foul language this time!" He grinned at me sheepishly.

"Good to hear."

Tips for Working with the Staff

1. Learn the names of your aides

Remembering the names of the nurses and aides who work with you goes a long way toward establishing a friendly relationship.

"I can't keep track of them," John admitted. "Actually, I don't even try. I just call them all 'Miss.'"

"That's a lot better than the other things you could be calling them," I teased, "but I think you'd get better service if you remembered their names."

"But there's so many of them! My memory ain't as good as it used to be."

"Well maybe you could just try keeping track of the main ones, like your day and evening aides, and the day and evening nurses. Don't worry about the ones who cover for vacations or the ones who are here when you're asleep."

"Yeah, I guess I could do that." He was saying yes, but his tone said no.

"I'm going to write the names down for you, and then you can use this paper to remind you."

He appeared relieved to have a memory prompt. "Can you tape it up on the side of my dresser? That way I can take a look at it when I'm in bed."

16

"Great idea. And I'll be sure to use tape that won't strip the finish, so we won't get any problems from the administration."

2. Be polite

It's the job of the staff to take care of the residents, and if you could do things yourself, you wouldn't be here, so it might seem unnecessary to thank the staff for doing their jobs. I've noticed, however, that staff members tend to respond better to residents who are polite and express appreciation for their help than to those who don't.

"So I said to her, 'Thank you, Loretta' and she started smiling!" John told me. "And then the next day she showed me a picture of her kids."

3. Bunch requests

I used to wait tables when I was in college and every so often I'd get a group of diners who, instead of asking me for everything they needed at once, would make a request and then wait until I'd returned to the table to put in another request. For me this meant an extra trip to the kitchen when I was already very busy. Similarly, if you can ask the nursing home staff for all that you need at once, it will save them time and effort. Some residents find it helpful to keep a notepad by their bed to accomplish this. As one resident joked, "By the time they answer the call bell, I've forgotten what I wanted. They love that!"

4. Find your compatible staff members

One of the good parts of having so many staff members at your disposal is that there is always someone with whom you get along especially well. Try to find a few of these people in your nursing home so you can work with them to get your needs met. For example, if you and your day aide have a strictly business relationship, she's not the person to ask to water your plants. Don't sweat it! Ask your night aide buddy or the friendly porter. And remember, if someone is grouchy with you, chances are excellent they are being grouchy with the person in the next room, and with their family at home. Don't take it personally. To quote a friend of mine, "They're not doing it to you, they're just doing it."

The Call Bell

"I had a really hard day yesterday," Mary told me.

Her face looked drained of color.

"What happened?"

"I got sick and nobody came to clean me up for over an hour."

"An hour! That's awful! Did you use your call bell?"

"No."

"Why not?" I was surprised.

"I didn't think it was an emergency."

"I know you don't like to bother people, Mary, but that counts as an emergency."

Every bed in every nursing home has a button to press to call the nurses and aides. Typically, it's on a long cord and clipped to the bedcovers for easy reach. When you press the red button, an alarm goes off at the nursing station, and a light goes on above the door to your room to notify staff you need attention. "Call bells" are not only for medical emergencies. Use them when you need care quickly, for example, when you've spilled juice all over your bedclothes. On the other hand, employing the call bell sparingly will reduce the noise on your floor, so try not to use it if you know the nurse is going to be by any minute with medication. You can also "bunch" your requests and the staff and your neighbors will appreciate your efforts.

One of the most common complaints I've heard over the years is that the call bell isn't answered quickly enough. I wish it weren't so, but yes, you're right, often it's not. There are many people working to educate staff members about this (including me). Given the current reality, the best suggestions I can offer are to plan ahead as much as possible, avoid busy times, and cluster requests. Also, if you find you need more care than you're getting, consider asking to change to a room closer to the nursing station. That way you'll have easier and more frequent access to nursing staff since they'll be passing by your room more often.

For people who have difficulty using the standard call bell due to physical challenges, there are other types of call bells available. To get one, I'd suggest asking the staff member who's easiest to talk to and who gets things done, whether that's your nurse, rehabilitation therapist, social worker, or other staff person.

You're always supposed to have access to the call bell, so if your aide makes a habit of putting it out of your reach, it's okay to say something to her, and then to the nurse, and up the chain of command until the problem is resolved.

Chapter 3

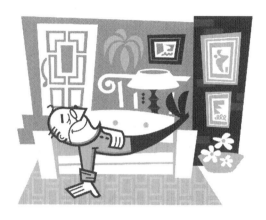

Managing Your Medications

Know Your Medications

If you're able to remember what medications you take, why you take them, and how much you're taking, you've made yourself a partner in your own care. You'll be able to say to the doctor, "When you increased the dose of medication X, I noticed side effect Y." Or, "When I had symptom Z in the past, medication A helped me."

Write Them Down

If you can't remember—not unusual, as residents are often on many medications with changing dosages—ask the nurse to write it down for you. Keep a notebook to write down any med changes and ask the nurse or doctor what side effects you might expect when starting and stopping medications or changing doses.

Vivian pulled out a black-and-white composition book from her drawer and handed it to me. "Take a look," she said. "I ain't letting no one give me nothing without keeping track of it."

On each page was the start date of the medication, both the trade name and the generic name of the medicine, and the dose and time the medication was given. "Viv, this is impressive! How did you know about the two different medication names?"

"That was messing me up for a while, until I learned that them long names were the ones from the scientists that made them and them fancy ones were the ones to try to get you to buy 'em."

"They make them sound so good, don't they?" I laughed.

"And they're pretty, too, some of 'em. But I ain't taking nothing ain't on this list, unless my doctor tells me first."

"I plan to do the same thing when it's my turn, Vivian, if I'm able to."

Count Your Pills

Another technique to keep track of your meds is to count your pills. Note, for example, that you get a little pink one and two big white ones in the morning and a blue oval in the afternoon. Believe me, if I have the wherewithal when I become a resident, I will be counting my pills every day, and so will all the retired nursing home staff. Observing which medications are given and at what time of day helps you keep track of side effects, ensures that you're taking everything you're supposed to and nothing more, and provides experience that makes it easier for you to handle your own medications upon discharge.

Side Effects

Every medicine has side effects, but that's not a reason to stop taking medication. As a matter of fact, sometimes a medication is prescribed for the side effects! It's important to talk to your doctor about what you're feeling after taking your medication because it's your body and you're the one that knows it best. A good approach is to tell the doctor your symptoms and let him or her make the diagnosis. One woman told me how she related a number of symptoms to her doctor, and on the way out the door she added, "Oh, and by the way, my elbow's been hurting me." This seemingly unrelated pain turned out to be a symptom and the key to her diagnosis!

Standing versus PRN Orders

Medications are prescribed as either "standing" orders or "PRN" orders. Standing orders are those medications that you'll get automatically when the nurse gives out medication at various points in the day. PRN orders refer to medication that's given "as needed" or "Pro Re Nata" in Latin. A helpful way to think of it is "Per Request of the Nurse." This means that you won't get the medication unless you ask the nurse for it. Pain medication is often prescribed this way to avoid it being administered if you're not in pain, as it frequently causes constipation. Sometimes I'll visit with an obviously suffering resident who tells me she didn't want to "bother" the nurse by asking for pain meds. It's not a bother! It's the job of the nurse to give PRN meds as requested, and it's the job of the resident to let the nurse know when you're in pain or need a PRN medication. If you're too shy or forgetful to ask for pain meds when you need them, consider talking to the doctor about switching to a standing order.

More on Pain Medications

"What do YOU want?" John asked when he saw me at the door.

"My goodness, you're usually so glad to see me! What's wrong?"

"I'm sorry," he said, rubbing his arm.

27

"I was up all night. My arm is killing me, and the pain medication isn't helping at all. Those pills are a joke. I won't even take them any more! I wish the doctor would give me something stronger."

"Here's the thing, John. How is the doctor going to know you need something stronger if you're not taking the pain pills he ordered for you?"

If you find your pain medication isn't working for you, it's important to let the nurses know. They'll report it to the doctor. When the doctor reviews your record, it will be very clear you need more pain medication if you are taking every dose ordered and still experiencing pain. It will be far less clear that you need stronger pain medication if you've stopped taking the medication that has been ordered for you.

Despite years of studies that show that pain in nursing home residents is routinely under-diagnosed and under-treated, doctors tend to be concerned about offering pain medication. There are some residents who ask for pain medications they don't really need, and perhaps doctors are wary due to this or due to the side effect of constipation. Pain is subjective. It's hard for other people to tell how you are feeling, so they have to take your word for it—or not. Your best bet is to calmly ask for a review of your pain medications. Some nursing homes have pain management specialists who can offer an expert opinion, if requested.

Every once in a while, pain medications cause **hallucinations.** Don't panic! They'll go away after the medication is stopped.

"I was feeling these bugs crawling on me," Vivian told me, scratching her arm at the recollection, "but I knew there wasn't no bugs. It was that medication they was giving me."

"How did you know?" I asked, because sometimes it's hard to tell what's an hallucination.

"There ain't no such thing as pink and purple bugs! And it started happening right after they added that pill. So I

*stopped taking it. Oh, they fussed! But I
refused."*

"That's your right, Viv."

*"I know. I read my "Residents'
Rights" pamphlet cover to cover! Once I
stopped taking the pill, the doctor can-
celled it, and them bugs went away."*

"So you're good now?"

*"Right as rain! And they gave me
something else for the pain."*

Palliative Care

Palliative Care, also known as **Hospice
Care,** has **pain reduction** as its goal. If you
are very ill, and perhaps close to the end of
your life, you might want to focus on improv-
ing the quality of your days by enhancing
comfort and reducing the unpleasantness
of undergoing further medical tests and
procedures. Studies have shown that many
people on hospice care live longer than
those with similar illnesses who aren't on
hospice. Most hospice programs accept
people who have about six months left to
live and give extensions when people live

longer than that.

You can talk to your doctor (and often your social worker or nurse) about whether you're a candidate for hospice care. You might be thinking you won't be around much longer and, by talking to them you find out that you have more time than you thought. That's good to know and will probably change your approach to your nursing home stay, and your life. Or perhaps you find out that you don't have much time left, and knowing that allows you to better decide how you want to spend your time.

Don't be shy about asking for information. Many people assume that if it were time for them to be on hospice, the doctor would have mentioned it. In fact, most physicians aren't so good about talking about dying. They're trained to help people get better, not to help people have a kinder, easier death when it's clear they're at the end of their lives. It's the hospice people who are trained to do that.

If your doctor agrees you might benefit from hospice, you'll be evaluated by the hospice nurse, and you can get more information about the program before making a commitment. It's okay to hear about the program and then decide against it.

People on hospice have a specially trained aide that is assigned to them several hours a day and treatment that focuses on making them comfortable. Some people get hospice care in the nursing home, while others move to a freestanding hospice center, and others receive care in their own homes or that of a family member, if that is financially and realistically possible. Hospice also offers support for family members, so this can be a way for you to help your family, even though you're in need of help yourself.

"I wasn't sure I was going to like hospice," Clarice was saying. "I'm almost 91, and I believe in heaven. I'm okay with dying, but I didn't want to dwell on it. Then I thought about my daughter. Evelyn's been through so much, losing her brother, and then her

husband. I couldn't leave her without some help."

"The hospice program has been helpful for her?" I asked.

"Oh, yes! She was worrying herself sick over me. Now at least I know she's getting some rest when the hospice aide is here taking care of me. And they have them counselors to talk to, so I know someone will be there for her after I'm gone."

"It must ease your mind not to be worrying about her worrying about you."

"I'm still a mother, honey, and I need to take care of my girl."

"It sounds like you're both taking good care of each other. It's heartening to see."

Chapter 4

Relationship with Your Medical Doctor (MD)

The MD's Schedule

Sometimes residents tell me, "I never see my doctor," and I know it's true. While there may be no face-to-face contact, your doctor still knows what's going on with you via the nurses and a monthly review of your care. If you haven't seen your doctor, it's because the nurses haven't noticed anything that would warrant a visit from the doctor. It's actually a good thing not to see a lot of the doctor!

If you need medical attention, the nurse will let the physician know.

How to Talk to Your MD

The Newspaper Headline Approach

When your doctor does come to see you, remember that talking to an MD is not like having a conversation with a regular person. In a normal conversation, one person asks how you are, the other answers, "Fine," and then the true exchange begins from there. If you tell your nursing home doctor you're "fine," he's on to the next room to see someone who needs his help.

Because the doctor is usually short on time, I recommend what I call the "Newspaper Headline Approach." Just like newspapers grab your attention by giving the most important information in the headline, so should you when speaking to your MD. When your doctor asks how you are, your answer could be the headline: "I'm in Pain" or "I Have Three Things I Need to Talk to You About." Then be sure to give the most pressing concern first. Keeping a written list of issues between MD visits can help you keep track of and prioritize your concerns.

MD Communication Book

You can also request to see the MD at any time. Most nursing homes have a communication book where messages are left for the doctor to read, and you can ask the staff to leave a message for the doctor from you in the communication book.

Medical Explanations

The MD will be the staff member who will tell you about test results and can best explain medication changes. The nurses can usually answer follow-up questions or offer further explanation.

The MD Orders Everything

Every medication, every therapy, every meeting with the psychologist, every off-campus pass is ordered by the MD or it's not allowed to happen. That being the case, there's no point in reasoning with a staff member that you've been taking an over-the-counter cough medicine, as needed, for 50 years and therefore you should be taking it now. All you can do is tell the nurse you'd like to see if the doctor can order your regular cough medicine or an acceptable substitute. On the one hand, it might seem silly, but on the other, your doctor knows the effect that cough medicine could have when combined with your other medications.

Willie grimaced and pressed his hands to his temples. "This headache is killing me. Sweetheart, open that drawer and get me some aspirin."

"You've got aspirin in there?"

"Yeah, and some cough syrup. Last time I had a cough it took them two days to get me something, so I had my grandson pick it up at the pharmacy across the street. Now I don't have to bother with the nurses."

"It's definitely annoying to wait for something you can get in five minutes across the street, but Willie—there's no way I can give this to you."

"Why not?"

"I'm not your MD. How do I know

what these medications will do when combined with your other pills? How do you know?"

"Well…" He paused.

"I wouldn't chance it, Willie. You're on a lot of pills. It's not worth it. Why don't you talk to the doctor? Maybe he'll order you the same medication, but at least he'll be able to track you to see if there are any drug interactions."

"Yeah, my wife said the same thing," he agreed halfheartedly. "I just hate waiting on those nurses."

"I know. There's a lot of waiting here."

We stared at each other for a moment, and then Willie reluctantly said, "Go ahead." He watched as I removed the bottles and threw them into the trash.

"Thanks, Willie. I'd have been wor-ried sick about you. I'll leave a note for the doctor telling him you want to see him."

"Ten bucks down the drain," he

grumbled. *"Well, at least you and my wife will be happy."* He rubbed his temples for emphasis.

"I'll see if they can get a phone order for some pain reliever so you don't have to wait so long."

Chapter 5

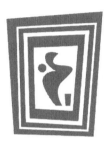

What Rehabilitation Can Do for You (and How to Do It)

83-year-old Nellie sat on her bed, telling me about a recent off-campus trip with her daughter.

"It was so nice! We walked down the street to that new restaurant. When I got tired, I just sat and rested on my walker." She pointed to the padded seat on her rolling walker.

"It's great you're able to get around, Nellie."

"You know, I couldn't walk when I first got here. And I didn't want to go to physical therapy either. I didn't even

want to get out of bed, but that girl from rehab made me, and now I'm glad she did. When I see those other people sitting around in therapy, not working, I just want to tell them to give it a try. Look what it did for me!"

Nellie's story isn't unique, but I'd like to see more people achieve her level of success. This chapter will help you make the most of the opportunity for therapy, so you know you tried your best, whatever the results.

What Is Rehabilitation?

Nursing home rehabilitation is made up of two main services—physical therapy (PT) and occupational therapy (OT). The goal of both is to help you regain physical functioning you may have lost after an illness, injury, surgery, or through lack of exercise.

Physical Therapy (PT)

The goal of physical therapy is to help you have as much physical movement and strength as you can. The PT staff members are the ones who will help you walk again, if possible.

In physical therapy, you'll have tasks like leg exercises from your wheelchair, standing, and walking between parallel bars. As you gain strength and balance, you'll begin using a walker and, perhaps, a four-pronged quad cane or a straight cane, until you can walk independently. Often the staff will have you practice on stairs so you can get up the steps to your home.

Occupational Therapy (OT)

The goal of occupational therapy is to give you the tools you need to engage in meaningful activities of daily living. Even though it's called "occupational" therapy, it has nothing to do with a paid job: it's about finding ways to do the things you need to do in life.

The OT staff will work with you to get your arms moving after a stroke, for example. They'll help you relearn how to brush your teeth, put on your clothes, and other essential tasks for an independent life. In OT, you might get trained how to use tools like a "reacher," which is a long metal stick with a gripper on the end that allows you to pick up things that are out of reach.

I leaned over to pick up the magazine that had slid off Miguel's lap while we were talking.

Miguel motioned for me to stop. "I got it," he said, nonchalantly.

I watched as he expertly grabbed the magazine with his reacher, raised it so he could take it into his free hand, and casually flipped it onto the bed. "Wow! You ought to be in the Reacher Olympics! You're great with that thing!"

Miguel smiled. "I've been practicing."

The Tasks of Rehabilitation

Mary was sitting very still, staring out the window when I came to see her.

"Are you okay?" I asked her. She didn't seem to have her usual energy.

She sighed, and said, "It's the rehab. I try to do what they ask me, but I just don't see the point." Frowning, she added, "Like today they had me moving all these pegs on a board. How is that going to help me get home?"

I smiled. "You know what they had me do after my bunion surgeries, Mary? Move marbles with my toes! I couldn't believe that was the exercise. It seemed crazy, but it did work."

"It did?"

"Yes, it did. Do remember the movie called The Karate Kid?" I asked her.

"It sounds familiar."

"Well, there's a boy in the movie who wants to become a karate master, and his teacher tells him to wax his car by moving his arm in giant circles to the left and to take the wax off the car in giant circles to the right. The kid gets angry after weeks and weeks of car polishing. That's when the teacher tells him that he'd learned important karate moves without realizing it. 'Wax on, wax off,' the teacher points out." I moved my arms in polishing motions. "That's what they're doing in rehab. All the peg-moving is helping you learn something *important, even though it looks like nothing much right now."*

Mary smiled. "Wax on. Wax off," she said, polishing an imaginary car in front of her. "Yes, I can see that."

In rehab, each meaningful activity is broken into small tasks. For example, sitting up in bed actually requires many actions: rolling to your side, swinging your legs over the edge of the bed, pushing yourself up with one hand, and maintaining an upright posture with your feet on the floor. When you master these small steps, you will be better able to carry out a larger purposeful activity. Try to keep this in mind when you're given what seems like a silly assignment. Keep your eye on the prize—getting better.

Pain Management

People occasionally find rehabilitation exercises painful. **Taking pain medications half an hour before a PT or OT session can reduce discomfort.** In general, though, rehabilitation can help manage pain. The

46

rehabilitation therapists have many "tools" in their bag of tricks to help reduce pain, including therapeutic massage, heat, cold, ultrasound, and interferential currency (IFC).

Therapeutic massage is done while you are fully clothed and is generally found to be very soothing.

Heat packs and ice packs can be applied on a painful area for relief.

Using ultrasound, the therapist generates increased blood flow and soothing heat by gently massaging a gelled wand or "sound head" on an affected area.

IFC involves putting pads on the skin and stimulating the nerve fibers with small, harmless, electric currents to reduce pain.

Often these rehabilitation tools are used together to provide the most pain relief.

Speech Therapy

Speech therapy can be an important part of the rehabilitation process for people who have difficulty speaking, for example, following a stroke or head injury. The training and exercises the speech therapist provides can result in major improvements in the ability to speak clearly. Speech therapists also provide training for people who are having trouble swallowing. Read more about that in the dietary department chapter (chapter 6).

Making the Most of Rehabilitation

Attending rehab is one of the most important things you can do soon after you arrive at the nursing home. The exercises will help you reach what is called your "maximum potential" in terms of physical functioning. The rehab staff will be working with you to become as independent as possible, and this can mean the difference between going home and staying in the nursing home for long-term care.

Go to rehab even if you don't think it will

help! Millions of people roll into nursing homes in wheelchairs and walk out, and it can happen for you. Give it all you've got!

Jerome came in on a stretcher and was so thin and frail that he looked as if he might be blown away by a strong wind.

"He's been bed-bound for almost a year," the rehab therapist told me, "but he's motivated and is making really good progress."

Every once in a while, I'd catch him working in the hallway.

"First your right foot," his therapist told him. Jerome moved his right foot slowly forward. "Good. Now your left." He dragged his left foot to meet his right.

I marveled at how difficult it seemed and then reflected on how long it takes to learn to walk the first time around.

Two months later, a small group of enthusiastic staff members gathered in the lobby to say goodbye to Jerome. I watched as he marched proudly out the door and climbed into the car waiting to take him home.

Use Your Depression

Many people feel depressed coming into a nursing home and with good reason—they're ill, not able to get around like they used to, away from home, dealing with lots of strangers, unsure of the future—the list goes on.

Psychologists often say that depression is anger turned inward. Anger is energy—and energy that can be used to fuel your rehabilitation. If you can, take your depression and turn it into anger. If you don't like the way someone treated you this morning, use the energy of your anger to take a few extra steps in PT in the afternoon. "Punch" your diabetes in your OT exercises. The more you get moving, the less depressed you will feel.

Finding Motivators

One good way to keep motivated is to find some friends in rehab who are going through the same thing that you are. Cheer each other on. You'll all appreciate the encouragement when a neighbor tells you, "You're making great progress."

Music is another good way to energize your rehabilitation. A 90-year-old woman I know used to listen to "light Italian opera" in her head while attending OT. I prefer the theme from Rocky, but use whatever works for you. If you have a CD, ask the rehab people if they'll play it for you.

I was impressed by the efforts of 81-year-old Frieda, who was training to use a prosthetic leg to replace the one she'd lost to diabetes.

"How do you keep yourself going?" I asked her. "So many people your age would have given up."

"I don't think about my age. I visualize walking out of here and going home."

And she did, with a boyfriend she'd met during her stay.

Don't Be Foolishly Independent

"So what happened?" I asked Willie, who was in bed, looking sheepish. "I heard you fell."

"That damn aide," he began and then stopped himself. "I had to go to the bathroom, and I got tired of waiting for her. So I tried to get there myself and I slipped."

I grimaced at the thought of his fall. "Are you okay? Are you in pain?"

"I've got a couple of bruises," he admitted, "and they gave me some pain medicine. But I'm more shook up." He shook his head slightly. "I really thought I could do it."

Every so often, I'll encounter a resident who, frustrated with having to rely on others for care, decides to walk without assistance against the recommendations of the rehab department. Very frequently the resident falls, leading to injury, a longer rehab process, increased monitoring by staff, and more frustration. I know it can be maddening to wait, but trying to walk or stand before being cleared by the rehab department is not worth it. They are experts in knowing when individuals are ready to move to the next level without harm. Their jobs depend on it.

If you feel you're ready to be more independent, ask the rehab staff to evaluate you. For example, if you believe you can ambulate around your room with a walker, the rehab staff will do an assessment, and if they agree, the doctor's orders will be changed to reflect this. That way you can move about your room with confidence, with staff consent, and without jeopardizing your health.

Maintaining Progress After Completing Rehabilitation

The rehab department will be able to keep you in training as long as you're making progress. Once you've reached your "maximum potential," you will graduate from rehab.

For short-term residents, discharge from

rehab is usually closely followed by dis-charge from the facility.

For long-term residents, many nursing homes have trained nursing assistants on your unit who will work with you after gradu-ation to retain the functioning you gained in rehab. They'll provide range of motion exer-cises, help you to stand, and walk with you in the hallway. If you find you're not getting assistance ambulating on the unit, for example, tell the nurse or social worker. Even if it's very busy, the nursing staff is required to carry out the doctor's orders in the chart, including orders for post-rehab maintenance exercise. It can be helpful for you to know if there's a doctor's order for you "to walk with assistance for fifty feet, twice a day," so you can keep track of things yourself.

Post-Rehab Adjustment

Completing rehabilitation can be a big adjustment, especially for residents who aren't going home. Days that were once focused around the rehab schedule now feel less purposeful. **It's important to find some new structure and/or focus in your life** to avoid becoming depressed.

Mary was lying on her bed, fully dressed, with her crocheted quilt not quite covering her feet. She opened her eyes when I knocked, and then closed them again, motioning for me to come in.

I closed the door to her room and settled myself in the chair by her bedside. "Mary, are you okay?" The recreation therapist had pulled me aside earlier in the day to tell me Mary hadn't been attending their programs recently.

"I'm just relaxing," she replied, and then sighed heavily. "I guess I got nothing to do but relax, now that they stopped my therapy."

"Oh." I nodded my head slightly with sympathy. "You 'graduated' from rehab. Did you get everything you wanted from it?"

Mary opened her eyes and fixed them upon me. "It helped some. I can't say it didn't. But I can only walk a few steps before I lose my breath, and I've got stairs going up to my house I can't manage." She sighed again. "They say I'm going to have to stay here, and I don't see any way around it. I can't get into my house, and I'd rather stay here than move back south by my sister. At least here my church friends can visit me."

"You'll stay connected to your people if you live here." Mary's room was filled with cards and flowers from church members, and her pastor came by almost every week. "And then there are the friends you've met here…the ones from the activities."

She gave me a sheepish look. "I've been feeling a little down. I haven't been going like I used to."

"So I've heard. They miss you down there!"

"They do?" She seemed surprised.

"Of course they do! You were a regular. The rec therapist is worried about

you, and she said some of the other ladies are asking about you."

"That's nice to hear." Mary smiled, slowly swung her legs over the side of the bed and sat up. "Maybe I'll go down again later," she said, and smoothed her hair.

"That would be great." I got up to look at the activities calendar. "They've got baking this afternoon. And there's lots of stuff going on in the mornings, now that your schedule is open." I started reading some of the activities out loud. "And there are even church services," I added.

"Oh yes, my church comes here every week. That's why I get so many visitors. I couldn't go down before because I was in therapy." She said wryly, "I guess the good news is that I can get there now."

Exercising on Your Own

Many residents ask their rehab trainers about safe exercises they can use on their own to supplement the work they're doing in rehab or to use after graduation.

I know a man who'd lost both his legs to diabetes and compensated for this loss by lifting weights until his biceps were finely chiseled. I also witnessed a group of residents who participated in an athletic competition in their area, wheel-chairing in a race with others with disabilities. It was an exhilarating and inspiring event that changed their perception of aging and disability.

Some nursing homes have exercise classes available to anyone who wants them, or classes could be started if residents request them (ask your rehab or recreation directors or raise the issue at the resident council).

Reevaluation for Rehab

Once you've graduated from rehab, there are a few situations that qualify for reevaluation by the PT/OT staff. If you've been to the hospital during your nursing home stay, you may be reevaluated to see if you'd benefit from more therapy. If you've had a fall or gotten sick, you may have had a change in "functional status" that warrants another round of treatment.

"Look at this," Leroy told me in our psychotherapy session. He shifted his left foot over an inch on the foot pedal of his wheelchair.

"Oh my gosh!" Leroy had been given a 50/50 chance of moving his legs again after spine surgery. He'd shown no sign of movement in the three months since the surgery, and we thought he'd never walk again.

"The other foot is even better," he said, easily moving it a couple of inches over.

"Leroy, you can move! Go show this to the rehab people."

Leroy's small movements were a "change in functional status" that allowed him to start rehab again and eventually walk out of the facility.

Progress, Not Perfection

Not everyone who wants to walk out of the nursing home is going to do so, nevertheless, significant, meaningful progress still can be made. It makes a big difference, for example, if you can transfer from your bed to the wheelchair and back or if you can use your tableware to feed yourself. These are important accomplishments that will improve your quality of life.

Vivian was smiling when I entered her room for our session. "What's up? You look very happy today."

"Honey, I did it!"

"Did what?"

"I learned how to roll over in my bed!"

For months, Vivian had been frustrated and uncomfortable, stuck all night in whatever position she'd been left in by her aides. "Hurrah!" I cheered. "That must make a huge difference for you."

"Honey, you have no idea! Now whens they clean me up, I can turn by

myself without them having to push me. Some of them ain't so gentle when it comes to turning," she pointed out. "Last night when I was tired of sleeping on my right side, it took me a while, but I flipped onto my left!"

Wheelchair Evaluations

The rehab staff evaluates the type of wheelchair you're using to make sure it fits your needs in a wide variety of ways. There are many different types of manual wheelchairs—some of which will allow you to wheel yourself, while some require others to push. Wheelchairs can have high backs for those who require additional support, while those who need more cushioning are sometimes given recliners, which are like chaises lounges with wheels.

The facility is responsible only for providing manual wheelchairs, but there are also electric wheelchairs, or "power chairs," with rechargeable batteries. The rider learns to operate a hand control (similar to a "joy stick" for video games) that directs the chair. Not every facility allows its residents to use power chairs, usually due to narrow hallways and safety concerns. Most people who have power chairs got them while in the community and/or paid for them privately.

The rehab staff will help find the best chair for you and will assess your vehicle as your needs change. If you're not comfortable with your wheelchair, it's important to let the rehab staff know. There are many reasons to have your chair and the assorted pads and accessories assessed. Perhaps you're finding yourself leaning to one side or the wheelchair is repeatedly heading to the left even though you're driving straight ahead. Maybe you'd be more comfortable sitting on a different cushion, or you need anti-tipping devices installed. There is something for almost every issue, so it's worth asking.

The Wheelchair Is Your Ride

Just as you'd take your car in for an inspection, keep an eye on your wheelchair to make sure it's in good repair. If you notice anything loose or wobbly, tell the staff so it can be fixed. Chairs are cleaned on a regular basis, but if you've spilled juice on it, it will need to be washed right away.

There are a variety of products to **make your wheelchair more useful and homey,** such as cup holders or storage pockets that hang over the side of the chair. You can ask your nursing home if they have any of these items, though these are generally accessories you'd need to buy with your own funds or ask for as a gift from a visitor.

There are also ways to make your chair more fun and to add a sense of humor to your ride. You can get a colorful chair or apply stickers or even order wheels that light up as you roll through the halls. I know one man who used his settlement money from a lawsuit to purchase a bright red motorized scooter, which he rode while wearing a black leather vest and dark sunglasses.

Chapter 6

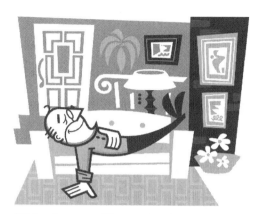

Dietary Department: Food, Glorious Food

Most nursing homes are cooking for several hundred people (including staff) from various ethnic groups and with special dietary needs. The chances are excellent that the food isn't going to be the type you're used to.

In every nursing home in which I've worked, I've encountered as many residents telling me how good the food is as there are residents voicing dietary complaints. As a foodie, I know I'm not going to be thrilled with my meals when I'm a resident, but I hope to use some of the following strategies to make them more palatable.

The Dietitian as Resource

The dietitian is responsible for making sure you have the meal plan that's right for you, such as a sodium-restricted diet or chopped food. Beyond that, the dietitian can review the menu with you and note your likes and dislikes. This information gets relayed to the kitchen staff and will be reflected in your food tray. You'll notice that your meal comes with a slip of paper. If you look closely at the paper it tells you what the meal is, and has a line for "likes" and "dislikes." So if you love mashed potatoes but hate gravy on them, tell your dietitian. If there's a food you're craving, it doesn't hurt to ask if it's served there—you might be pleasantly surprised.

Use Condiments

Find diet-compatible spices and condiments to spruce up your meals. For example, one sodium-restricted lady I know swears by Mrs. Dash. A food service director who's eaten at the nursing home for 25 years ("How would it look if I didn't eat my own food?") uses hot sauce. Depending on my dietary restrictions, I plan to have a smorgasbord of seasonings to take to the dining room, including sesame seeds, oregano, and flavored salts. I'm going to have a little spice caddy on my lap as I'm wheeled to the dining room!

Chopped and Pureed Food

Sometimes people aren't able to swallow regular food and are prescribed chopped or pureed food. If you're on a chopped or pureed diet, take heart; it doesn't mean you'll be on that diet forever. Many have swallowing difficulties that improve with training from the speech therapist. She'll give you exercises to strengthen the muscles in your throat, like sticking out your tongue or repeating certain sounds. While they might seem strange, they do work.

In the meantime, if it's hard to sit at a table with folks eating regular food while you've got puree in front of you, ask the nurse, dietitian, or social worker if you can switch to a table with other people eating pureed or chopped food.

"What is that?" Nellie asked me, eyeing the lunch tray her aide had just placed on the table in her room.

I looked at the plate, and then turned to the paper sticking out from under the tray. "It says it's roast chicken." We stared at the scoop of chopped, light brown food for a moment.

"Maybe if I pretend it's chicken salad…"

"Great idea!" I replied.

Thickened Liquids

Prior to working in a nursing home, I'd never heard of thickened liquids, and they are probably new to you as well. Adding a thickener to liquids makes it easier to swallow and can prevent choking. Thickeners with different consistencies are used (honey-thick, nectar-thick, pudding-thick), depending on the degree of difficulty you have swallowing. Thickener can be added to liquids—such as coffee—to make them drinkable, or pre-thickened liquids might be offered to you. If you've been prescribed thickened liquids, remember:

Speech therapy can help improve the ability to swallow, which often makes the liquid restriction temporary.

Drinking liquids that are actually supposed to be thick—or imagining that the liquid you're drinking is a shake or smoothie—can help make them more palatable.

Residents with swallowing difficulties, or dysphagia, often have colored wristbands to alert staff of their needs. You might find staff members checking your wrist before they offer you a beverage to make sure they don't serve something potentially hazardous.

Resist the temptation to drink regular liquids if thickened liquids have been prescribed in order to reduce the chances of getting aspiration pneumonia, which is when fluids go down the windpipe instead of the esophagus and cause an infection in the lungs.

"Sweetheart, could you get me a cup of water, please?" Willie asked me when I walked into his room for our psychotherapy session. "With ice," he added.

"Willie, aren't you on thickened liquids since you came back from the hospital?" I looked for his armband. The sliver of color sticking out from his shirtsleeve confirmed my suspicions. Willie was hospitalized with a stroke last week and had just returned a couple of days ago.

"Yeah, but I don't like them." He wrinkled his nose.

"Nobody really does, but were you told about the risk of aspiration pneumonia if you're not ready for regular fluids?"

70

"Yeah…what is that again?"

"It means the water could 'go down the wrong pipe' and end up in your lungs. Then you'd have to go back to the hospital."

Willie closed his eyes for a moment. "I don't want to go back there."

"I don't want you to either." I'd been relieved when Willie'd returned to the nursing home in good condition. "You're getting speech therapy, right?"

"She just left."

"Well, give it some time. It works wonders." I took a stern tone. "And don't be asking people for water before you're ready. What if someone doesn't know you can't have it, and you choke on it? That person would feel awful!"

"Alright, Sweetheart, don't get upset now." Willie tried to calm me.

"I'd feel awful if something happened to you."

"I know you would."

Home-Cooked Meals

If you have friends or family members who cook, ask them to bring in meals as a gift. If you have several people who can do this once a month, you can stagger your requests so you're getting a home-cooked meal once a week. The dietitian may even be able to arrange to have this food chopped or pureed in the kitchen, if needed.

If you're on a pureed diet, ask your family to bring you pureed soups and other foods that are meant to have the consistency of puree, like puddings. Check with your dietitian to be sure you are brought meals that follow food guidelines.

Eating Out

Nursing homes often take off-campus trips to restaurants, and I plan to sign up for every one of them when it's my turn to be a resident. I'm also hoping my friends and family take me out to eat on occasion or bring in takeout food. I expect I'll use most of my **P**ersonal **N**eeds **A**llowance (PNA) on ordering in food.

Unless things are significantly different in your nursing home than in the ones I've worked in and heard about, don't plan on having leftovers the next day if you leave your extra food overnight in the communal refrigerator. I don't know why this happens—and it shouldn't—but it seems that there's a 20% chance of leftovers making it back to their rightful owner.

"I was so disappointed," my aunt told me over the phone from her assisted living in California. "I had these wonderful leftovers in the refrigerator, but they were gone when I went to get them for lunch today." She sounded crestfallen.

"Isn't that terrible! The same thing happens all the time here too and has happened at every nursing home I've ever worked in."

"It does?" She sounded surprised. "I thought it was just me."

"I don't know if it's good or bad news, but it happens all the time," I told her. "The only consolation is that it's

Eating in the Dining Room (Versus Your Bedroom)

I know when I'm a resident, there will be some days I'll just feel like hiding in my room; nevertheless, there are good reasons to eat in the dining room with the other residents.

You can meet some people you like and have a pleasantly social meal.

Even though tables might be "assigned," you can request a seat with someone whose company you enjoy and create or expand a friendship.

Because **the nursing staff will be in the dining room with you,** you'll be able to get better service than when your tray is dropped off in your room, and you're left alone until someone comes to pick it up.

seriously bad karma to take things from nursing home residents. Remember what Bea Arthur used say in her TV show Maude? 'God'll get them for that!'"

My aunt laughed, and I could tell some of the sting of the affront had left her.

Food Rotation

The menu in nursing homes is set many months in advance, and it changes every week. Week one provides a certain set of meals, week two another, and so on. My dad grew up on a one-week food rotation. He knew Monday meant spaghetti and Tuesday was meatloaf day. He was happy with this. I, on the other hand, crave variety (except for Fridays, which is dumpling night). I'd like to see a four-week food rotation in nursing homes so I'd be getting the same meal only once a month.

Food Committee

Many nursing homes have a food committee made up of residents and led by a food service staff member. Other nursing homes address resident food concerns as part of their resident council meetings. The group provides a forum to discuss residents' food concerns and helps to plan menus for special holiday events. It's a great way to get involved, meet other residents, and contribute to the creation of a food plan you enjoy.

"Again with the Cluck-Cluck"

Yes, nursing homes serve a lot of chicken. I can't deny that. One resident added some humor to this fact by her memorable comment, "Again with the cluck-cluck." If all the chicken is getting on your nerves, remember that alternatives are available for every meal. There are usually two options, plus an alternative, plus sandwiches and, perhaps, even a salad platter. Ask for what you want!

Menus

The menu for the week should be posted prominently on your floor or unit. Ask a staff member to point it out for you. You can also request a copy of the menu.

Weight Loss

If you're overweight, your dietitian can help you choose a weight reduction diet. I highly recommend this because being overweight (in addition to being unhealthy) has a huge impact on your level of mobility. I've seen people begin to walk again, or manage to wheel their own chairs, after losing weight. If losing weight allows you to change from a two-person transfer to a one-person transfer, it could mean the difference between permanent nursing-home placement and returning home. This is because many insurance companies cover only one home health aide, so unless a family member is available, someone requiring two people to get out of bed in the morning will be unable to manage at home. The dietitian will help you lose weight at a safe, gradual pace.

Whether you're over your desired weight or not, the staff will let you know if you're losing weight faster than is recommended (two pounds a week maximum). Weight loss of more than ten pounds in a month will trigger the staff to monitor your intake very carefully. The nurses, aides, and dietitian will increase the frequency of your weigh-ins, and encourage you to eat. You might be referred to the psychologist or psychiatrist, since over- or under-eating can be a sign of depression.

"The nurses asked me to talk to you because they were worried about you. They said you'd lost a lot of weight recently," I told Ms. Pisani, who frowned at my comment.

"They won't leave me alone! Eat! Eat! Eat! That's all I hear!" She banged a frail hand against the arm of her wheelchair.

"It's like having 20 moms, isn't it?" I gently teased her.

She smiled slightly.

"So why aren't you eating? Is it the food or that you're not hungry?"

"I just don't feel like eating. My son comes and brings me food from out-side, and I eat a little of that and I'm full." She shrugged.

"Try to do the best you can because they're going to keep bugging you until you start gaining weight." I nodded toward the can on her table with the straw sticking out. "You've been drinking those shakes?"

"Sometimes. They're not bad with ice."

"Good. Those will help put the weight back on." Ms. Pisani nodded, but I got the sense she wasn't as concerned as she should be.

"You've lost 20 pounds since you came here, Ms. Pisani, which is a lot in a short amount of time. Sometimes if people keep losing weight quickly, the doctor recommends a feeding tube. Do you know what that is?"

"A feeding tube? That doesn't sound good." Ms. Pisani was more attentive.

"It's good if it saves your life," I pointed out. "Sometimes when people aren't eating well on their own, they are fed through a tube that goes into their stomach. It doesn't hurt, and it's

79

temporary, but I'm sure you'd like to avoid that if possible."

Ms. Pisani looked shocked. "Absolutely!"

"I don't mean to scare you," I said, "and I don't know what your exact medical situation is. I can tell you that it's really important to eat even a little bit at a time and get your weight back up on your own if you can."

"Thank you for telling me. I don't want a feeding tube." She picked up her nutrition shake and took a sip.

I smiled. "Now that's a good start."

Chapter 7

Social Work Department:
The Social Worker Is Your Friend

Most of the nursing home staff focuses on attending to your physical and medical needs. It's the social work department, along with the recreation department, that focuses on your emotional needs. The social workers in a nursing home are in charge of an astoundingly wide variety of tasks. While the exact duties can vary slightly from facility to facility, the social work department is generally one of the busiest in the nursing home. This chapter will give you an idea of what social workers can (and cannot) do to help you.

Initial Settling In

The social worker will visit you to offer emotional and practical support when you first arrive at the nursing home, and they'll check in with you periodically thereafter. This is a good time to ask questions about any concerns you may have because your social worker can provide information and talk to other members of the treatment team for you. You can also ask the nurse and other staff members to contact the social worker if you need to talk to her.

If you're at the nursing home for a short-term stay, the social worker can explain the process so you know what to expect as you go along. If you're planning to stay long-term, she can help you make the facility feel like home by assisting you with tasks such as getting a telephone installed or having your mail forwarded, if there's no one in the community to help you with these undertakings. Busy as she is, she can't run to the store for you, except in rare instances out of the goodness of her heart. For most errands, it's best to rely on a friend or family member.

Psychosocial Assessment

Early in your nursing home stay, many staff members will be getting to know you. They'll be coming by your room to ask questions that will help them to assist you. The social worker's questions in particular will be quite personal—about your family, your schooling, your mental health history, etc. It's important to give a clear and accurate snapshot of your life so the team will have a sense of the supports available to you and the areas in which you'll need help.

"So I told her, they's going to ask you a lot of personal questions." Vivian was recounting how she'd advised her new roommate, who'd just arrived the night before. "But don't let that scare you. They asks them of everybody. How's you gonna get the help you need if you don't tell them?"

"If I remember correctly, Viv, you weren't so happy about all those questions." She'd nearly chased me out of the room the first time I met her.

"Oh, I hated them nosy questions! At first I thought, what they got to know about my daughter for? She ain't talked to me in years. But then I thought, they's got to know so's they can call her if something happens to me." So far, this was the most Vivian had revealed to me about her daughter Margaret, whose name was on the contact sheet of her chart but who had yet to make an appearance. "We's had our troubles, but she's still my daughter."

Room Assignment

The admissions department will set up your initial room placement, though you can talk to your social worker if you and your room-mate are having a difference of opinion over, say, the temperature of the room. The social worker can help resolve complaints or find a new room if necessary. If you become a long-term resident, it's likely you'll have to move from a short-term or rehab floor, and the social worker will help find a room that will be right for you. Often you'll be able to visit the floor beforehand, so you can choose between rooms.

When dealing with an interpersonal challenge, it can sometimes seem that "the grass is greener" elsewhere.

Willie was tense when I came to visit him. "What's the matter?" I asked.

"It's that guy outside my door." He gestured toward the hallway. "He's driving me nuts!"

"You mean the guy that's clapping all the time?"

"Yeah, and laughing out loud at nothing. I've got to get off this floor. Maybe I'll move to 2," he pondered.

"Yeah, but on 2 there's that lady near the nursing station who calls out all the time."

"Mmmn." He nodded with recognition. "Well, I don't want 3 because that's the dementia floor. And on 4 most of the residents don't speak English. Maybe 5."

"That floor's pretty good, except for that grouchy guy with the loud voice."

"Oh yeah. I don't want to be around him. I guess I'll just stay here. It's really not that bad."

I've had conversations like this one on every floor in every nursing home in which I've worked.

Private Rooms

Many, if not most, residents prefer to be in a private room, but these are often limited in number. You can ask your social worker to be put on the list for a private room, though keep in mind that it's likely to be quite a while before one opens up. Nursing homes will offer private rooms to those on the waiting list; the rooms, however, are also needed for residents who have an illness that could be contagious or have behavior issues, habits, care needs, or medical equipment that might be disruptive to a roommate.

If you're on the list, keep in mind that the wait will feel more like waiting for the seasons to change than waiting for the bus.

Keep yourself busy while you're waiting, and get out of your room and off your floor, if possible. If you have a roommate whose company you enjoy, revel in the companionship.

"Are you going?" I heard Mary ask her roommate, the frail Ms. Pisani, whose appetite was still only fair. "They'll have cake and music. It's real nice," Mary said enticingly, though Ms. Pisani seemed hesitant. "I'm going. We can sit together."

Ms. Pisani looked at Mary gratefully. "Okay, I'll try it."

The recreation therapist had been watching this exchange, waiting to push their wheelchairs down the hall. "Wonderful!" she said. "You'll like it. The performer is great, and we're going to have red velvet cake today. Mary always comes down, don't you, Mary?"

"Whether I'm up to it or not. There's no sense sitting around alone up here."

Family Contact

The social worker is usually the main contact person with your family during your stay. I say "usually" because, as with other areas of care in a nursing home, who is in touch with your family can depend on individual circumstances and the personalities of the staff members. Sometimes the charge nurse on the floor can be very involved with families or if there is a language barrier between the social worker and your relatives, another staff member will step in.

In general, though, the social worker will be in touch with your family to discuss things like room changes, clothing needs, advance directives, financial concerns, etc. She can help arrange a pass to go off-campus over the holidays and at other times during the year. The social worker will also invite your family to your Care Plan meeting, where they can meet with team members to discuss your care.

Care Planning

At Care Plan meetings, members of the treatment team will join together to discuss your needs in great detail. These meetings are the single most important time for your family to be at the nursing home because the team will be sitting together with pen and paper (or computer) to discuss what is and isn't working with your care. Changes will be put down in black and white, and the staff will focus on meeting these new goals.

Residents are allowed to be at this meeting. In some nursing homes, they are strongly encouraged to attend. When I'm a resident, I intend to be at every Care Plan meeting I can muster the strength to attend. I'll want to know what the treatment team is doing for me!

"So I went to that meeting," Willie was saying to me. "And it kind of freaked me out."

"In what way?" I asked him.

"Well, at first I was like, wow, they know everything about me." He nodded

his head. *"I was impressed."*

"You didn't think they knew as much as they did?"

Willie chuckled. "I had my doubts."

"So what was the freaky part?"

"Well, then I was thinking, my God, they know everything about me!"

We both laughed. "No where to hide, huh?" I joked.

"They even knew about those medicines I had in my drawer."

"It wasn't me, Willie," I protested. "Once we threw them away, and you promised to stop taking them, I didn't tell. Maybe the porter did after he emptied the garbage."

"I think it was my aide. She keeps an eye on me pretty good," he said with appreciation.

Advance Directives

Some of the tougher stuff to deal with needs to be addressed at this phase of your life. Those who have advance directives in place seem to be calmer and feel more in

Advance Directives

Advance directives include:

A Living Will, which is a statement of your wishes for your care if you're unable to say what you want, and it is especially helpful when you don't have a health care proxy.

A Health Care Proxy, which is someone you trust to carry out your health care wishes. It's important to talk to your proxy about what you do and do not want in terms of medical care.

A Do Not Resuscitate Order (DNR), which states that in the event of cardiac or respiratory distress certain medical treatments won't be performed.

A Durable Power of Attorney (DPOA or POA), which is someone you trust to make financial decisions and to carry out tasks like paying bills and going to the bank for you.

control of their situations.

Your social worker will give you more information about each of these, as laws and forms are different in each state. There are "in hospital" forms and "out of hospital" forms, which can confuse even the most savvy resident and family members. The social worker will help you fill out the forms and make decisions about your care. This is also a good thing to discuss with your psychologist because it can be an emotional process.

I could tell by Vivian's furrowed brows that she was worried about something. "What's up?" I asked her.

"That new social worker just left. She was asking me about who I want to be my, my lawyer, or something…"

"Your power of attorney?"

"Yes, that's what she called it! My POA, she said." Vivian bit her lower lip. "You knows I don't like to talk about Margaret." Margaret was Vivian's only child. She hadn't spoken to her in

years, and she rarely mentioned her in our sessions. "I'd like for her to be my POA, but that don't make no sense. I know that. She don't even call. It's just wishes."

"You wish for things to be different between you and her."

"I sure do." Vivian sighed. "But it just ain't that way, and it ain't gonna change in the next few months. I needs to take care of myself, and find someone else."

"Do you have anyone else?"

"Well, there's my cousin Lois, but she ain't too good herself. I guess I could ask her son—the good one, not the other one—if he could help me. We's always had a nice relationship."

"He lives nearby?"

"Not too far. He comes to see me 'bout once a month." Vivian seemed to settle her mind. "He's a nice boy. He'd do that for me. I used to care for him when his mama was at work some-times."

"I'm glad you have someone to help."

Burial Funds

While we're talking about the tough stuff, I might as well bring up the issue of burial funds. Most people in nursing homes are on Medicare and Medicaid, and in order to qualify for Medicaid, you have to have a specific relatively low amount of money in your bank account. The exact amount depends on what state you live in. The money you set aside for burial, though, doesn't count toward that amount. It, therefore, makes good financial sense to put away money toward your burial fund if you're in the situation of "spending down" to become eligible for Medicaid.

A lot of people don't want to think about this when they first come to the nursing home, which is when they're most likely to be in the period of "spending down." Most people don't want to think about dying, I've found. I was, therefore, very inspired by an 86-year-old woman I helped briefly when I worked in a senior apartment building.

"When I die," Anna said to me, matter-of-factly, "I'm going to be buried

upstate with my brother and his wife."

"You've planned this out already?"
I asked.

"Oh sure! Honey, you've got to pre-pare as much for death as you do for life. Maybe more, because you'll be dead longer than you'll be alive," she pointed out.

"You're right!" I said, surprised that the logic of this hadn't occurred to me before.

Shortly after this session, we both decided she didn't need therapy any more. Anna made more sense than most people I'd met inside and outside of long-term care.

While putting your affairs in order can be challenging, the social worker will help you with each step, including setting up a burial fund. You might want to think of this as something you're doing for the people you'll leave here on earth. It's a gift to them to have planned out and paid for much of your service, relieving them of some difficult decisions and financial burdens at a time when they'll be grieving your loss. It's a gift to you as well, because it can be a huge relief to know that you're taken care of even after you're gone.

A few weeks after her ninety-first birthday, Clarice asked me to get out a pen and paper. "I want you to write this down and give it to my daughter when I go."

"Okay," I said, pulling out my pen and holding it above a small stack of clean white sheets of paper. I often take dictation for residents, though I wasn't sure what Clarice had in mind.

"I'd like the following songs to be sung at my funeral," she told me. "They're my favorites."

She proceeded to list five hymns, singing a few lines as she told them to me.

"Those are lovely, Clarice. I'm sure they'll be a great comfort to your friends and family."

"It's a comfort to me to know they'll be sung. Now put that in my chart, okay?"

"Okay, and I'll make a copy to put here on your bulletin board." I gestured toward the wall. "Clarice, do you think you'll be going soon?"

"Pretty soon. I know I won't be reaching 92, and that's fine with me. I'm ready."

Financial Benefits (Medicare/Medicaid/SSI/Veteran's Benefits)

Many residents enter the nursing home under their private insurance and need help getting the paperwork together to file for the additional benefits they're entitled to, such as Medicare, Medicaid, Social Security Income, and Veteran's Benefits. Many other residents have Medicare but not Medicaid. The social worker will work with you and your family on the paperwork, along with the business office at the nursing home, to send out your applications. Having the paperwork done correctly and swiftly helps

both you and the nursing home, which nat-
urally wants to maximize the amount it's
paid for providing services.

*Ms. Pisani was crying when I
entered her room for our session. "Ms.
Pisani, what's wrong?" I asked her,
alarmed. I was hoping she'd begin to
feel better after getting to some activities with her roommate, Mary.*

*"The social worker just left," she
said, blowing her nose into a tissue and
then adding it to the growing pile on her
tray table. "She said I have to go on
public assistance." She sobbed and
reached for another tissue. "I've never
needed help from anyone! Me and my
husband always managed to get by,
and now look at me!" Tears streamed
down her face.*

*"Ms. Pisani, I'm sorry you're going
through all of this," I told her, closing her
door and sitting down beside her.
"Lots of people feel the way you do, but
maybe it will help if I explain something."*

She looked at me expectantly, dabbing her eyes with a tissue.

"When you say, 'public assistance,' you mean Medicaid, right?" I asked her.

She nodded "yes."

"Most people here have Medicaid. As a matter of fact, 95% of all the nursing home residents I've ever met have been on Medicare and Medicaid."

"They are?" Ms. Pisani asked, her eyes widening with astonishment.

"Oh yes. You're in excellent company." I smiled. "That's just how things are done. People come into the nursing home on Medicare or private insurance and pay for some of their care with their own funds until they run out of money. Then they go on Medicaid and pretty much everything is covered by Medicare and Medicaid after that."

"I didn't know…" Ms. Pisani had stopped crying.

"Most people don't. It's not the greatest system, but you're not alone, and there's no shame in it. It's just the way it

is. In a way, you're lucky."

"What do you mean?"

"Well, at least there are benefits for you to collect, and you know you'll be taken care of for the rest of your life. People of my generation, at the end of the baby boom, have been putting money into the system our whole lives, but who knows what will be there by the time it's our turn to go into the nursing home." I shrugged. "All I can do is sock a little money away and not worry about it now."

"I guess I have it made, then, don't I?" Ms. Pisani joked.

"Made in the shade...." I replied.

Going Off-Campus

In an ideal world, your kids could call up and say, "Ma, we'll be there in half an hour. Get your coat ready." They'd whisk you out to your favorite restaurant and bring you back late or even the next morning. In reality, even an excursion of a few hours requires an order from your doctor.

Frustrating, I know, but physicians are responsible for determining whether you're in good enough health for the trip—it's their licenses on the line. Fortunately, once they've determined that you are, they can write an order reading something like, "May go out on pass with responsible party," and then you don't have to go through the process again (unless there's a change in your medical condition or a new doctor).

Be aware that the "responsible party" is someone listed in your chart with contact information. If you'd like to leave with someone else, you'll probably need to have permission from your contact people.

If you're planning to go out of the facility, your family should contact the social worker, who'll work with the team to make sure you have MD orders, medications, and transportation, if necessary. It's especially important to plan this ahead of time during the holidays, since it's likely to be a busy period with many people going out on pass.

As I entered the unit, I heard yelling at the nursing station and caught a glimpse of Willie wheeling himself down the hall at a brisk pace, his face flushed with anger. I followed and poked my head in the door of his room.

"Am I glad to see you!" He gestured for me to come in. "These people are messing with me!"

"What happened?" I asked, sitting on the edge of his bed since his chair was piled high with packages. Ribbons and birthday wrapping paper streamed over the cushion and onto the floor.

"My cousin came up from Virginia for my birthday, and we were going out to the movies. We were going to the 4 o'clock show."

I glanced at the clock. It was 4:15 p.m.

"I know, I know. It's too late now. They wouldn't let him take me out! They said he wasn't in my chart. I got so angry, I told my cousin to leave." Willie shook his head. "The nurse wanted to

call my wife to ask her permission! Ask my wife! Can you believe it? Like I'm a little kid or something!" His foot bobbed up and down on the footrest of his wheelchair. "I'm a grown man, and I'm not asking my wife's permission for anything."

"I can see your point, Willie. That would mess with your relationship." Willie's wife visited regularly and brought him home-cooked meals several times a week. Despite his confinement to the nursing home, it was Willie who called the workmen to take care of the household tasks at their home that he still considered his responsibility.

We sat in silence for a moment. "You know why they do that though, don't you?" I asked him.

"To embarrass me?" His foot was still bobbing up and down. "I know, it's a legal thing."

"Yes. While you're here, the nursing home is legally responsible for you. Once someone signs you out, that person becomes legally responsible. Of course, you and I, and even the nurses at the desk," I said with humor, "know you can decide that your cousin is perfectly fine for you to go out with. But what about Mr. Jackson?" Mr. Jackson was a very pleasant though extremely confused man who lived down the hall from Willie. "What if someone the staff didn't know showed up and said they were taking him out?"

Willie sighed, and his jiggling knee became still. "I see what you mean," he admitted. "Jackson would go off with anybody."

"The rules are designed to protect the Mr. Jacksons of the nursing home world, but unfortunately the Willies of the world get caught in the protective net too." I looked at him sadly. "I'm sorry you missed your birthday movie."

"Me too." His foot bobbed again for a moment and then stopped. "My cousin's leaving town tomorrow, but he's coming back in a few weeks, and we're going to *try again. I'm gonna have the social worker put him in the chart."*

Discharge Planning

The treatment team, led by the social worker, will make sure your discharge home is a safe one. If you've come to the nursing home for rehab, the discharge process will begin after your rehabilitation is complete. Sometimes people need to apply for Medicaid in order to be able to fund their home care, and that process (at least in New York State) can take several months. In that case, your discharge will swiftly follow its approval. As part of the process, the social worker will arrange home care, if necessary, and get the supplies you need to make your place livable, such as a walker or a commode.

If you want to transfer to another nursing home, or to assisted living, the social worker is there to help you. If you need to find an apartment, room, or house, however, you'll have to rely on a family member or a friend, because searching for an independent home is hard to do when you're a nursing home resident, and it's beyond what the social worker can do for you.

For more on discharge planning, see chapter 13.

Mental Health Care
(Psychology and Psychiatry)

 Psychology

Entering a nursing home is very stressful and can shake even the most well balanced individual. The social worker may be able to offer some support with this stress, and it can be very helpful to see the psychologist. Of all the people working in the nursing home, the psychologist is the only person whose job is to sit and speak with residents privately for an extended period of time on a regular basis. Sessions are generally once a week for about 20 minutes. The psychologist won't be sent to see you unless one of the team members thinks it would be helpful. It's perfectly fine for you to be the one to ask for the service.

Even residents with supportive family and friends can find it helpful to talk to a professional about the changes in their lives and how to cope. Sometimes there are things residents would prefer not to discuss with their family members because they're private or out of concern for worrying or overburdening them. Sometimes residents want to discuss their family and how their illness is affecting their relationships. Frequently, residents need information and assistance in figuring out how to live in this new environment. A psychologist, who knows the staff and the nursing home system, is often able to help in a way that family members are not.

While the psychologist will have to write notes for each session, the notes do not generally contain personal details, so that your conversations are as confidential as possible. If privacy is something you're concerned about, be sure to address this with your psychologist.

Psychiatry

Sometimes people find that their moods are helped by antidepressants or other psychotropic (mood-affecting) medications prescribed by the psychiatrist. Psychiatrists are medical doctors who specialize in mental health issues and the medications to treat them. They meet with residents who arrive at the nursing home already taking psychotropic medications and those the team thinks might benefit from them. The meetings are generally brief and might occur every three months, more often if necessary.

If you are experiencing feelings of depression, there are many things you can do to help yourself feel better, and you can discuss your depression with your psychologist. But if after talking about it and trying to take some positive actions, you find yourself still feeling blue and lacking the energy to follow through with the psychologist's recommendations, it might be time to consider talking to the psychiatrist. An antidepressant can be like a "jump start" to get you going again so you can begin to take positive steps on your own. The medications don't work as quickly as jump-starting a car though. You can expect it to take about three weeks to feel the positive effects of antidepressant medication. People often take antidepressants for a while until their lives become more balanced, and then they work with the psychiatrist to gradually taper off the medication.

Chapter 8

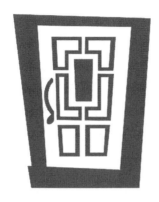

Lodging Complaints

Resident's Bill of Rights

You probably got a list of "Resident Rights" when you were admitted into the facility. If you're like most people (who find themselves overwhelmed when they first arrive), you didn't feel up to reviewing them at the time. Chances are they're still in your top drawer; if not, you can get a new copy from your social worker. They're also posted in the hallway, and they're worth reading.

As a resident, you're entitled to a certain level of care, respect, privacy, and freedom. The details of this are outlined in your "Resident Rights," which vary in exact details from state to state. It's here you'll discover that you have a right to refuse medications if you don't want to take them or to voice complaints through the ombudsman's office, described below.

I recommend reading through your rights. It can be an enlightening and empowering experience.

Ms. Pisani was in tears when I arrived. "What's wrong?" I asked her, as she dabbed her eyes with the tissue I'd handed her.

"They can do whatever they want to me," she sobbed. "I can't even say anything!"

"What do you mean? Did something happen?"

"Yes!" She put her fragile hand to her chest to soothe herself. "I had a shower today, and afterward, the girl left me there with just a sheet—a thin sheet! I was freezing!" She shuddered and pulled her sweater tighter around her neck. "She didn't come back for half

an hour, and I didn't dare say anything."
She gave me a searing look. "I've heard
what they do if you speak up for yourself." She began to sob again.

I sat with her quietly as she cried
and then said gently, "You read about
something bad happening to a resident
in the newspaper, right?"

"Yes."

"The paper is full of all sorts of terrible things, Ms. Pisani. But I know the
people here, and they really try to do a
good job, most of them. You're allowed
to talk to them about how you're feeling
and to try to work it out."

"I could never do that!"

"Have you heard of the Resident's
Bill of Rights?"

"It's the staff that has all the rights!"
she exclaimed.

"Funny, the staff members say the
same thing about the residents. They
think you guys have all the rights!" I
smiled. "The Resident's Bill of Rights
says you're allowed to speak up for

yourself without having to worry about something happening to you because you did." I leaned toward her. "But really, there are ways of letting your aide know what makes you uncomfortable without even getting into that. Would you like to hear a way to handle that type of situation?"

"If you think it would work," Ms. Pisani said. "I don't want to be left like that again!"

"Well, we're going to need to use some psychology on your aide, okay?" With her assenting nod, I continued. "Before your next shower, mention to her that you get cold very easily, and ask her to bring a warm blanket or something she can wrap you up in. Then, when she does this after your shower, be sure to thank her and tell her how wonderful it was. Make a big point of it, like it's the best thing that happened all day."

Ms. Pisani giggled. "I used to do that with my husband when he washed the dishes! What a fuss I made!"

"Did it work?"

"Like a charm." She giggled again. "I could try that. I used to be quite the actress!"

Working with the Staff

Your job as a resident is to work with the staff in the business of your health care, the daily task of getting you up and ready to face the day. That's right: Reports of your retirement have been greatly exaggerated!

You and your aides will get into a routine—they'll know how you like things, and you'll know how they work. At first, though, the routine will be unfamiliar and might seem strange and uncomfortable. **All the interpersonal skills you used at work and other social situations will come in handy** here.

Mr. Watson was a heavyset man who was lying in bed with his right leg elevated. He clicked off the television when I knocked on his door and explained the reason for my visit.

"They told you about me, huh?" he asked. "I figured someone would show up about that."

"I was told you were angry, but I wasn't given any details," I replied. "Can you fill me in?"

He launched into a lengthy, expletive-filled description of his morning care routine. It was clear that he and his aide weren't clicking. "I told them to get me someone else," he said angrily. "I don't need to put up with Diana's nonsense!"

"I see," I told him, and paused for a moment before continuing. "This might seem like a funny question, but I'm wondering what kind of work you did for a living." The chart had said he worked in a factory.

"I was a supervisor at a car parts factory. Why?" He looked at me suspiciously.

"Oh, a supervisor! You had to handle a lot of personalities in that job!"

"Oh sure, but that wasn't a problem. It was just part of my job. This here, this is different. I'm sick! I should be taken care of!" His face reddened with anger.

"Ideally, yes. But people are people and there are a lot of personalities here too. I'll bet if you used some of your supervisor skills, you'd have them eating out of the palm of your hand."

"But…but…" he stammered.

"I'll bet you were really good at it. The chart said you worked there for 25 years."

"I was good at my work, yes," he admitted.

"Just think about it, Mr. Watson. I'll check back with you next week to see how things are going."

The following week, I was surprised to see Diana straightening up Mr. Watson's room when I came by to visit.

"I thought you were going to change aides?" I asked Mr. Watson when Diana had left the room.

"I was, but I thought about what you

117

said. I had to apologize to her for cursing at her. She's really a nice girl, once you get to know her."

"Yes, she is." Diana was always pleasant and friendly, and I could talk to her about the residents.

"Yeah, I'm actually going to miss her," he said, sounding surprised by this. "I got my discharge date. I'm leaving in two weeks, after we get a ramp for the front of my house."

"Good to hear, Mr. Watson. A short and sweet stay."

"I don't know about sweet, but I'm glad it was short."

The Chain of Command

Like most organizations, nursing homes have a hierarchy. If you're having trouble resolving a problem with someone or something at one level, you can address it on the next level. For example, if you're unable to work things out with your aide, you can turn to the nurse for assistance. If you're having trouble with the nurse, you can ask to speak to her supervisor, and so on up the chain of command.

Nursing homes strongly prefer you allow them the opportunity to settle problems in-house, rather than turning to outside agencies. Most problems can be sorted out within the nursing home structure because the chain of command works in your favor. Nursing homes desire happy residents, contrary to reports you might have heard. They'll do their best to address your concerns and meet your needs. If you've exhausted all possibilities, however, there are people outside the nursing home to help you.

Ombudsman

A long-term-care ombudsman is a resident advocate who works through your State Unit on Aging. You may have seen your ombudsman in the facility talking with the residents. Though they visit regularly and the staff knows them, they are not part of the nursing home staff. If you have concerns, the ombudsman can listen and offer suggestions and, with your permission, share your concerns with the nursing home to help you resolve complaints.

State Department of Health

Long-term care is a highly regulated industry, and the regulations come from the State Department of Health. One rule every nursing home must follow is that the complaint hotline number be posted in a location visible to the residents and their families. A call to "The State" will trigger an outside investigation into the problem. One of your rights as a resident is being able to have complaints investigated without fear of reprisal (retaliation). A call to The State is likely to ruffle some administrative feathers, so it's best to reserve such a call for situations that can't be solved within the nursing home.

Chapter 9

Your Belongings

Leaving Your Old Home Behind

For most people, the shared quarters of a nursing home room requires leaving most of their stuff behind. This can be challenging, especially if you didn't get a chance to say goodbye to belongings acquired over the course of a lifetime. Let yourself acknowledge and grieve this loss and give yourself time to adjust. Keep in mind, however, that **you are more important than anything you accumulated along the way.** You still have you.

As I wheeled her to her room, I noticed Ms. Pisani was holding a photo album on her lap. "Do you mind if take a look?" I asked her, as we settled in her room.

She handed me the album, and we spent some time talking about the photos of her family before I gave the album back to her. She clutched it tightly and said, "My sister-in-law just brought it over. It's all I have left of my home."

"You've decided to stay here?" Ms. Pisani had been debating whether or not she could manage at home.

"Yes. They're clearing out my house today. I wish I could be there, but…" She gestured toward her thin, bandaged legs and her feet in blue Velcro-strap hospital shoes. "I can't make it in this condition." She bit her lower lip. "I hope they're careful with my things. I collected a lot of good furniture over the years." She paused for a moment, reflecting, and added, "I had a nice

home."

"I'm sure you did. It must be hard to let it go."

"Yes. It is. But what can I do? It's too much for me now, and I can't fit it here."

We looked around the small area she now called home. "No, I suppose you can't," I agreed.

"Besides," she said, "I'm donating most of my things to charity. They should be able to make some good money from them."

"What a wonderful idea! How nice to know your things will be put to good use!"

"As my mother always used to say, when life gives you lemons, make lemonade."

Making Your Room Home
It's worth the effort to add a few homey touches to your room. You'll feel better in a room that's more personal, and it will give the staff the chance to see you as a full and complete person, and to get to know you.

Creating a New Home

A nursing home room can hold the basics, and yet it can also hold so much more if you let it. I love walking into rooms that give me a sense of the resident's life, filled with photos and mementos. While your choices depend on the size of the room and your access to your belongings, here are some of the things I've seen used to create a home:

Framed photos

Plants

Fresh flowers

Plastic flowers

Vases

Paintings

Calendars

Artwork
(sometimes created
in the recreation
department)

Framed diplomas
and other awards
and certificates

Small tables

Small chairs

Bedspreads
and quilts

Doilies

Clocks

Books

Telephones

Computers

Communication
devices

Small refrigerators
(depending on the
nursing home)

"If your house is being cleaned out today," I said to Ms. Pisani, "is there anything else you want here besides your photo album? Maybe there's something small, but important, you could bring here for a touch of home."

"I hadn't thought of that," Ms. Pisani said. "I was so focused on the fact that I had to leave…"

"Lots of people are. But it's not all or nothing. If this is your new home, you deserve to have it feel homey. Is there anything you'd want here?"

She was quiet for a moment. "My sister made me a needlepoint picture— years ago, way before she died—and I'd love to be able to look at that." She smiled. "It would make me feel like she's watching over me if I could see that picture here."

"That sounds like a lovely idea. Can we call the people clearing out your house and let them know? I can do it right now if you'd like." Within minutes, it was arranged.

125

Letting Go

Sometimes people go into the hospital and then the nursing home following a fall or some other sudden event. They never expected to be leaving their home and never got the chance to say goodbye to it. If this happened to you and you find yourself thinking of home often, you might want to find a way to say goodbye. This could be through prayer, talking about or writing about your home, or whatever way you have used in the past to heal from loss (besides time). Some people might find it helpful to try the following mental exercise:

In the relative comfort of your nursing home room, close your eyes and imagine yourself once again in your home. Imagine yourself walking from room to room, saying goodbye to your belongings and thanking them for their service. Allow yourself to cry if you feel like it. Release your belongings to provide service for someone else in need. Allow yourself to feel gratitude for this day, for your life, and for your strength and resilience.

Labeling Clothes

*"They're stealing my clothes,"
Willie informed me the minute I entered
his room.*

"What happened?"

*"My wife bought me three new
shirts—nice ones, too, like I told her,
and they never came back from the
laundry. Those laundry people are
thieves!"*

"Were your shirts labeled?"

"What?"

*"Did your wife bring them to the desk
to get your name and room number put
on them? Because otherwise the laundry staff have no idea whose clothes
they are."*

*"I don't know. I'll have to ask her."
Some of the steam seemed to have left
him.*

*"We can check the lost and found in
the laundry room." I reassured him. "My
other theory on missing clothes is that
stuff that's supposed to be in room 103
is hanging in the closet of room 301 or*

Willie Jones' clothes are in Wally Jensen's room because the numbers and names are so similar."

"That's true," he acknowledged. "I found someone's pants in my closet the other day."

"Not everyone here is going to realize they're not wearing their own pants or be able to say something if they notice," I pointed out. "We'll tell the nurse and do a search. In the meantime, make sure anything new gets labeled. It might still get lost, but if it's not labeled, it'll get lost 100% of the time."

The person or department responsible for labeling varies depending on the facility; every nursing home will have someone in charge of this important function. They'll also re-label your clothes if you have a room change, so expect that your clothes will be missing briefly while this is being done.

Clothing Attrition

Despite the efforts of you, your family, and

staff members, it's reasonable to expect you're going to lose some clothes along the way. It happens in the best of places, simply because there are so many people and so many clothes. I know it's very frustrating and disheartening, especially when you don't have much and clothes are expensive and hard to come by; nevertheless, it does occur. Depending on the circumstances, nursing homes might reimburse you for missing items, especially if they've been logged in the records as being among your belongings.

When things "go missing," I find it helps to remember that it's not happening just to you. It doesn't take away the loss, but it does make it sting less to know you are not alone.

Clothing Store

Because it's difficult, and sometimes impossible, for residents to get out and purchase new clothing, most facilities have a traveling clothing store come into the nursing home twice a year. The clothing company transforms a common area of the building into a department store, bringing in clothes, shoes, hats, coats, watches, jewelry, and other accessories.

Residents can go down and pick out what they want, and the money comes out of their account at the nursing home. If you are unable to make it to the clothing store, nursing aides will generally assess your needs and choose items on your behalf. The clothing store will alter items if necessary, and they'll be sent for labeling before they come up to your room.

It's a good idea to save some money for these events because it's a great opportunity to shop without having to rely on family or friends. Be aware that the prices tend to be higher than what you might find if you were able to go bargain shopping due to the convenience of the store coming to you and providing alterations. The clothing store also offers the kind of fabrics that can withstand the hot water of the heavy duty washing machines in the nursing home, so that you'll get more use out of these sturdier clothes.

Lock It Up

Some residents prefer to have their most important items in a locked drawer in their room. If your room doesn't already have a locked drawer, ask the nurse or your social worker to get a lock put on your dresser drawer. The maintenance department will install a lock and give you the key. Some residents put the key in their pocketbook, knapsack, or a bag kept on their wheelchairs. It's best not to put it in your pocket because if an aide is helping you with your clothes at night, it's easy for the key to get lost. You won't be able to check your pockets in the morning because the clothes will be off to the laundry room.

Chapter 10

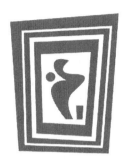

Your Money

A Money-Free Society

It might feel strange—after a lifetime of making sure you've got some cash on hand—to leave your pockets empty, but the reality is you are largely freed from money when you live in a nursing home. Your daily needs are being met by the facility, and there's nothing much to buy. If there's something you want to purchase in particular, you can withdraw money from your nursing home bank account or ask your social worker to withdraw the funds for you. It's best to take out money as you need it, rather than leave cash lying around. That will be one less thing to worry about.

John was frantically searching through his pockets when I showed up at his door.

"I can't find my money!" he exclaimed. "I usually have it in my shirt pocket, but it's not here!"

"How much is missing?" I asked him.

"Twenty dollars. I always keep a twenty in my pocket, just in case." John received fifty dollars a month as his Personal Needs Allowance, so twenty dollars was 40% of his monthly income. Relatively speaking, this was a huge amount of money to lose.

"When was the last time you saw it?" I asked.

"Last night." He stopped short. "I had a new aide last night! I'll bet it's still in my shirt pocket!" His face fell. "But my shirt's in the laundry."

I made some phone calls and dis-covered the laundry staff had found a crumpled twenty-dollar bill in the dry cycle. A quick trip to the laundry room and back reunited John and his cash, which he promptly stuck back in his shirt pocket.

"John," I said, with some humor, as I began my talk on relative income, locked drawers, and changing old habits. "Didn't we just go down this road?"

Personal Needs Allowance (PNA)

Most residents will be eligible for a Personal Needs Allowance (PNA), which is a small sum allotted to you after Medicare and Medicaid pay for your nursing home stay. The amount varies depending on the state in which you live. In New York, for example, residents have received $50/month since 1980, which is about average for PNAs.

The PNA is generally used for items not covered by your nursing home stay, like clothing, haircuts, special trips, magazine subscriptions, preferred toiletry items, take-out food, gifts, etc. It's not a lot of money, and it takes skill to budget accordingly.

"I want to send Margaret a present," Vivian told me, *"and I needs your help."*

I'd long ago created a personal policy not to do special favors, in order to prevent job burnout, but I was flexible around favors that brought families together, especially families that had been estranged. "What did you have in mind?"

"I want to send her $120, 'cause I knows she needs it, but I don't want to send cash, 'cause I don't trust the mail."

"That's a lot of money, Viv! More than two month's salary! Are you sure?"

"I been saving," she told me. "Ten dollars a month for a year. I can afford it—see." She pulled out the notebook she used to keep track of her medications and flipped to the back. There, to my amazement, was a list of her funds and expenses, from haircuts to vending machine runs to money saved for Margaret.

"Wow, Viv! I've never seen anything like this in a nursing home before!"

"I knows what I'm doing," she said proudly. "I been raising myself since

I was 14. Now how can I send this money to Margaret?"

With help from the business office and the recreation department, I was able to mail out a birthday card with a hefty check to her daughter.

Bank Account

Your Personal Needs Allowance will be deposited into an account in the nursing home, unless you decide to have your family receive the money for you. Sometimes in the busy and overwhelming period following admission, the information that there's a PNA and a bank account gets lost. If you're reading this and wondering about your finances, ask your social worker whether you're eligible for a PNA and whether there are funds in your bank account.

Nellie poked listlessly at the chopped food on her plate. "I sure am tired of this!" She'd been on a chopped diet for weeks following her stroke. "My daughter usually brings me food from home, but she's been away."

"Why don't you order in some take-out?" I asked. "You could get some soup or yogurt or something that fits with your diet."

"I don't have any money," she told me, shrugging her shoulders.

"Really? I thought you got Medicare and Medicaid."

"I do."

"Well, then you might have money in your account downstairs, unless it's being sent to your daughter to buy you stuff."

"I don't know. Maybe they told me about it when I got here, but I was pretty sick, and I don't remember much from back then." Nellie had come a long way from when she'd been admitted. The nurses had told me they didn't think she'd make it, and now she was one of the more active residents. Her recent stroke had slowed her only briefly.

"Let me check," I said. "I'll be right

back." I left her room to make a call to her social worker and returned a few minutes later. "You've got over $1000 downstairs," I told her. "You can definitely buy some takeout if you want it."

"What!" Nellie smiled broadly at her newly found fortune. "How can that be?"

"You get $50 a month for your personal needs and you've been here for twenty months without touching your account, plus interest, so it's waiting for you at the bank downstairs."

"My goodness! Wait until my daughter hears about this!"

Check with your nursing home about banking hours. The bank is generally open many times during the week, with a schedule that accommodates people whose dialysis program takes them out of the facility several days each week.

Chapter 11

Recreational Activities: Having Fun in the Nursing Home

Socializing

One of the best things about being in a nursing home is the **opportunity to meet people and become part of a community.** As I mentioned in the introduction to this book, the nursing home is a world unto itself. The other residents you encounter are your neighbors. The staff members are your coworkers in the job of getting you up and ready to face the world each day. The connections you make within the community can transform the experience of your stay.

It was hard to find Mary in her room these days, now that she'd started attending activities again. I rushed up to her floor just after lunch, when I thought she might be getting her medication before the afternoon's recreation began. I spied her by the med cart and waited for the nurse to finish before we headed to her room.

"Did you hear?" she asked, smiling broadly.

"Hear what?"

"I was voted Resident Council President!" she beamed at me proudly.

"Congratulations, Mary! That's wonderful!" The role was highly regarded at the nursing home, representing the voice of the residents in various affairs. "I'll bet you'll be great at that."

"I'm really looking forward to it." She looked at me nervously. "You know, I'm feeling more like my old self again, and I've been pretty busy lately…" She trailed off and looked at me.

"So you're thinking it might be time

to take a break from psychotherapy?"

"Yes," she said. "Is that okay?"

"Of course it is. I was thinking the same thing too. You've come so far since we first started meeting, and I'm always around if you need me again," I reassured her. "I take it as a good sign when I can't find the people I'm looking for because they're in activities!"

Attending Activities to Reduce Depression

There's a theory on depression that suggests people who are suffering from it stop doing the things they enjoy, and because they're not participating in enjoyable activities, they become more depressed. In order to reverse this downward spiral, they have to push past their lack of energy and motivation and attend activities even when they don't feel like it. Once they start doing something interesting and fun, it gives them a little more energy to try the next event. The resident begins to reverse the downward spiral and starts to feel better again.

Seven Suggestions for

It can be challenging for adults to share space with an unrelated person. (Let's face it—sometimes it's challenging to share a home with family members and others we've actively chosen to be in our lives!)

In the nursing home, we're often exposed to people from unfamiliar cultures or with habits different from our own. On the one hand, this can be an exciting opportunity to talk with new types of people and expand your horizons. On the other hand, when folks are feeling ill and are in a new environment, they are not at their best and need some time to settle in.

Here are some tips to ease your adjustment and make the most of the opportunity to live in a community with others:

1. **Find friends** who live on your floor.
2. **Participate in recreational activities** provided on your floor.
3. **Get off your unit as much as possible** by attending activities open to the whole nursing home or spending time on the patio or in the lounge.

a Successful Stay!

4. **Go on off-campus trips** with the recreation department, and talk to your family about going off-campus with them, if possible.

5. **Sign up with a wheelchair-accessible transportation service** such as Access-A-Ride in order to make off-campus travel easier. Talk to your social worker about this.

6. **If there are troublesome residents on the floor, give them plenty of space** and enlist staff members for assistance. It's better to move out of their way than to engage.

7. If something needs to be fixed in your room (.e.g., light bulb replacement, creaky doors, etc.), **ask the nurse, aide, or other staff member to write down any maintenance needs for the maintenance staff.** There's generally a log book or some other system to keep track of necessary repairs.

"Willie, how come I always find you sitting in your room?" Willie seemed to spend a lot of time watching movies and reorganizing his dresser drawers.

"Where else should I be?" he asked defensively. *"It's MY room."*

"There's nothing wrong with spending some time in your room, but there are lots of other things going on here. Have you made any friends?"

"Friends!" he snorted. *"I can't talk to these people!"*

"Funny. I talk to people sitting in their rooms by themselves all the time, and I think they'd get along great if they found each other." I glanced at the recreation schedule. *"There's a Men's Club meeting this afternoon. Have you ever been there?"*

"I don't feel like going to a Men's Club." He picked up a DVD from his tray table. *"My grandson got this for me. I'm going to watch it today."*

"Can you do me a favor?" I asked him.

146

"What's that?"

"Can you watch the movie after you go to the Men's Club?" I gave him my most winning look. "I think the men are going to be viewing some old boxing matches together."

"Maybe next week. I don't feel like it today."

I sighed. He didn't seem like he'd budge at all. "So next week, then?" I scanned the calendar. "You'll like this, Willie—there's a Motown group coming! I've heard them. They're really good." I smiled at him. "Please!"

"Okay," he relented. "For you." He smiled back.

The next week I ran into Willie in the elevator on his way back from seeing the entertainers, chatting with some other residents and the recreation therapist I'd spoken to about getting him to the Motown program.

"Sweetheart, you were right! They were good!" He nodded toward the man on his left. "This here's James. We lived

a few blocks from each other before we got here." He looked at James. "We go back a ways, don't we, buddy?"

"Oh, yeah!" James smiled. "I've known Willie for years."

The two of them laughed at some shared joke, and I tried to picture them as younger men. "How great that you're neighbors again!"

Recreation Staff

The job of the recreation staff is to help you find meaningful ways to spend your time at the nursing home. Some of the activities might be solo pursuits, such as needlework, reading books, or listening to books on tape, and many will be recreation programs run by their department.

The recreation staff will help you find activities you enjoy and assist you in getting to the programs. The staff knows many of the residents, so if you're looking for someone who shares your passion for baseball or gardening or travel, let a staff member know that you're interested in meeting like-minded people.

Activities Calendar

Every nursing home has a calendar of events, generally posted in each room and in a prominent location on the floor. It's a treasure trove of possibilities! Take some time to read through the calendar or have someone read it for you. I recommend trying everything at least once and planning to attend at least one activity each day. People tend to do better with structure, whether they're in a nursing home or not, and scheduling activities is a good way to give your life some structure.

Transportation

Recreation staff will transport you to and from the activities, if needed. Most residents require assistance getting to the programs, so you're in good company if you need a lift to the events. Because the transportation can take some time, it's the ideal opportunity to chat with neighbors or take along some reading material.

The nurse called me to the desk when I arrived on the floor. "Can you see John today? He got mad when the rec therapist didn't get him for program right away."

John was still fuming when I knocked on his door. "I sat for half an hour waiting for a ride to that concert! I really wanted to see it, but how long can I wait?"

"The traffic can be bad, I know, especially with popular events. I think of it as running into a traffic jam on the way to the city," I said, with a note of humor in my voice.

He looked at me and laughed. "Hitting traffic, huh?"

"Yep. It drives me crazy, too. If I were a resident, I think I'd have to bring along one of those Seek-A-Word puzzles or some knitting or something, just so I could stay calm."

"That's a good idea. I'll bring some crossword puzzles next time."

"I'm glad to hear you'll try it again."

"I've got nothing but time. But I don't like to waste it."

Modified Activities

"Bowling!" Ms. Pisani said with surprise when I read the afternoon's events off the recreation calendar. "How is an old lady like me supposed to lift a heavy bowling ball?"

"They change the way you bowl, so almost everyone can do it. It's pretty cool. They'll either use a ramp you can direct toward the ball or it will be virtual bowling." I described the virtual program's use of a remote control, TV screen, and the image representing Ms. Pisani on the screen. "It's hard to imagine but worth checking out just because the technology is so amazing."

"What will they think of next?" Ms. Pisani mused, and I realized she was teasing me because of my gushing enthusiasm for the program.

Seven Suggestions for

As a psychologist, I often talk to wonderful people in their rooms who tell me there are no residents for them to talk to. It's not true! You're just not finding each other. Here are some suggestions for how to meet people you will like, even if they're not like you:

1. **Observe** the people on your floor to see who might be aware and able to carry on a conversation. Look beyond appearances because those who are in reclining chairs or seem very old or ill might be more alert and able than you'd think.

2. Try sitting next to them or asking an aide to seat you next to them and pose a neighborly question, such as whether they're enjoying the food or like the nursing home. **Allow some time for a relationship to develop.**

3. If they don't seem to hear you, **ask a staff member to help** seat you by their "good ear," if they have one.

Socializing Success

4. **Attend activities** that are likely to appeal to the most alert residents, such as ones developed around trivia games or current events, and try the same observation and connection skills you used with residents with rooms on your floor.

5. **Speak up in groups** so people get to know you, and if it's appropriate, say a little bit about yourself, like where you're from or your hobbies or past work. This can encourage other residents to share similar information and make connections.

6. **Ask the recreation and social work staff to help** you meet other residents who share common interests both in formal groups and outside of them.

7. Because it can be challenging to get together with residents you like due to mobility issues, **ask your family to assist you** in visiting with your new friends.

While not every program involves sophisti-cated technology, many activities have adjustments made so that people of all ages and disabilities can enjoy them. Aside from larger print in books, puzzles, and games, there are many kinds of adaptive equipment available. Talk to your recreation therapist about activities available at the nursing home and how you might be able to engage in the pursuit despite physical limitations.

Suggesting Activities

Most recreation directors are open to suggestions about the types of activities available. If there is something you'd like to do that's not already on the schedule, talk to your recreation staff member or to the director.

Creating Activities

Do you have knowledge or a talent you could share with other residents? Consider running your own activities. There are nursing homes where staff members assist residents in running Bible study classes, book groups, and other programs. Some of these are ongoing groups and other times they're special one-time events. The recreation staff will help your neighbors get to the program, and assist as needed. Resident-run activities are a great way to meet people, keep your mind sharp, and continue giving back to the world. Talk to your recreation staff about this.

Chapter 12

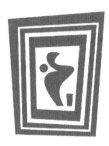

Family

Room-Warming Party

Encourage your family to visit you by hosting a room-warming party. Invite all your friends, neighbors, and relatives for an "open house." I know in theory you shouldn't have to ask, but sometimes it helps to extend the first invitation and to set a positive tone.

"I'm having a party!" Nellie told me at our next session. "That's right. My daughter got mad that no one came to visit me while she was away, so she said she'd make them come to see me."

"What do you think of that idea?" I asked, a little concerned about the attitude behind it.

"I think she's right." She grinned. "And I like parties."

"Great. Are you going to have it in here?"

"We talked to the recreation director, and she said we could use the dining room. We've got it all set up. We're going to have pizza and cake, and all sorts of people who I haven't seen in a long time are coming!" Nellie was buzzing with excitement.

"It sounds like fun. I hope you take lots of pictures."

Delegate Responsibilities

Even though most of your needs are being met by the nursing home, there's still some help required from family members, especially if you're managing or selling your home. It's very common for one relative to be doing more than others, a situation that sometimes troubles residents. If you can, help your family share responsibilities. For example, a long-distance relative can help with phone calls or email, while a local family member might be the person bringing home-cooked meals. If you've run out of your favorite toiletries, it's easy for families to order them on the computer and have them shipped to you, making it a task that can be delegated to anyone with an Internet connection and some funds.

Sometimes a request from you can be easier to hear than one coming from siblings. You're the best judge of your own family, so if you notice an imbalance, sometimes you can be the one to restore some caregiving balance.

"Is Nathan coming to this party?"
I asked Nellie. She hadn't mentioned her son at all.
"He'll be there. He's the one paying for it," Nellie informed me.
"Really?" I was surprised.
"Yes." She laughed. "Pamela was mad at him too, because he didn't come

to see me. So I told him he could make it up to her if he offered to pay for the party. He can afford it," she assured me. "He's got a good business."

"Did that make Pamela feel better?"

"Not completely. But it helped a lot." She shrugged. *"I'd have paid for it myself out of all that money I found in my account, but I thought it was better this way."*

"You're probably right, Nellie."

"I am. I know my kids."

Off-Campus Trips

Every so often, I'll encounter a resident who tells me they have no plans to leave the facility during their stay. "When I leave," they tell me, "I want to walk out that door and never come back." It's a legitimate viewpoint, though residents seem to fare better when they get out and about. I highly recommend getting out of the facility on every possible occasion, whether it's a resident trip, a visit home, an impromptu stroll around the block, or some time spent on the patio. Leaving the nursing home provides a refreshing change of scenery and reconnects you to the larger community and other parts of yourself.

"I ain't gonna be here next Wednesday," Vivian informed me.

"Okay, we can reschedule for another day. Where are you going?"

"Margaret be taking me out to lunch." She looked at me expectantly.

"What! That's awesome! What happened?" Aside from the money Vivian had recently sent her daughter, they hadn't communicated in over two years.

"She got my check and called me. We had a good talk. Things still ain't perfect, but good enough that we can have lunch together." She straightened out the rings on her fingers. "I ain't been outta this place since I been here, except to see the doctor."

"Oh my gosh, Viv! You're kidding!"

"I wish I was, but it's true. I don't even know what it's like to be outside

anymore. I've never been out in no wheelchair." She looked uncomfortable; her usual bravado had left her.

"Ahhh," I said softly. "People tell me it's a little strange at first, but just fine if you keep the focus on yourself and what you're doing."

"I'll be fine," she said, bravado returning. "The most important thing be's that I'm talking to my daughter again."

"Yes, that's the most important thing. And congratulations to you for making that happen."

"I knows I had to make the first move," Vivian told me. "My daughter be's a stubborn woman. I don't knows where she gets it from!" She chuckled at her own joke.

Holiday Planning

The holidays can be a challenging time to be in the nursing home, despite the efforts the staff takes to make it as special as possible. Most residents want to spend their holidays with family members yet don't want to be ones to bring up the subject out of fear of pressuring their families.

"Do you have any plans for the holidays, John?" Christmas was only three weeks away.

"Nah. I'm sure something will come up."

"What have you done for the holidays in the past?"

"When I was young, we used to go to my grandmother's apartment, but lately I've been going to my niece's house. She's got a couple of kids." John hadn't had many guests during his stay, but I'd seen photos of some children tacked to his bulletin board.

"Did you know you can get a pass to go off-campus? The doctor has to order it in advance, and your social worker will help set it up." I didn't want him waiting for visitors who never arrived.

"I can? They will?" John's eyes brightened.

"Yes, so you might want to talk to your niece about Christmas. It's not that far away."

His eyes dimmed. "I can't ask her. I don't want to be a burden."

"Maybe you're a joy and an important part of the family tradition," I suggested. Seeing that didn't meet with enthusiasm, I continued. "What if you asked her if there was something you could get her children at that craft fair that's coming up? That would give her an opening to talk about holiday plans."

"Yeah, maybe I could do that. I've got a few bucks I could spend on the kids." He glanced at the photo of the youngsters wearing matching coats and hats.

"And if you can't get to their house, maybe they could come by to visit some time over the weekend."

Advance Directives and Other Difficult Decisions

Talk to family members about the hard stuff —Power of Attorney (POA) decisions, Health Care Proxies, Do Not Resuscitate (DNR) orders, burial plans, etc. For more on these issues, see the social work chapter (chapter 7). By beginning these difficult discussions, you can gain more control over the situation and help your family through the process.

Clarice lost more weight every week. Today when I went by to see her, she was in bed, quietly reading her Bible.

"Hi, Clarice," I said, while the hospice aide got ready to leave for the day. "How are you doing?"

"I'm dying, Honey, but it's okay. I've got everything in place. All the papers are signed. My daughter knows exactly what I want." She held her hands on her Bible as she spoke.

"And Evelyn, how's she taking things?" I knew Clarice worried more

about her daughter Evelyn than she did herself.

"I think she's getting used to the idea. I don't know what else I can do to prepare her."

"No, Clarice, I think you've done everything possible. You've been a great power of example, handling this the way you have."

"Thank you, Honey. I try." She held out a frail hand, and I grasped it in mine. She giggled. "My goodness, your hands are freezing!"

"Clarice, I've had 103-year-old ladies warming up my hands for me!"

"Cold hands, warm heart," she said, as she rubbed some warmth back into me.

 Taking the Lead

You have a very important task in life right now. You're a role model for your family on how to handle aging, illness, and, at some point, dying. You don't have to do it alone, though. There are many people available in the nursing home, including clergy, the social worker, and the psychologist, to help you cope with these issues so you can better fulfill this life task.

Vivian looked radiant when I saw her the following week. "I got a load off my mind," she told me. "Margaret's gonna be my Health Care Proxy."

"She is?" I had hoped Margaret would be more involved with Vivian's life now that they'd reunited.

"I knows, she hasn't been around. But we had a good talk. I told her I needed her and that I wasn't gonna be around long."

"You're not?" I was dismayed to hear this.

"Well, I'm not gonna be here another 84 years! And I needs to get all my ducks in a row." She grinned at me. "Margaret was the biggest duck."

I laughed and, at that moment, realized that some of Vivian's radiance was due to a new hairstyle. "Hey, you got your hair done!"

"You like it?" she said, touching her hair. "Me and Margaret went to the beauty parlor after lunch. We had us a good time."

Chapter 13

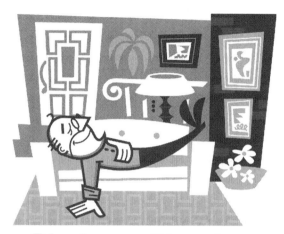

Discharge Planning: Homeward Bound

"I want to go home," Miguel informed me. *"What's taking so long?"*

"Aren't you still in rehab?" I asked him. *"It hasn't been that long."*

"It's been over a month! I've got to get out of here!" He ran his hands through his longish hair, leaving it sticking out every which way.

"What did you do in rehab today?"

"I walked down the hall and back." He gestured to show me how far, and then he continued to say, *"And then we went up and down that little platform*

with the steps."

"Steps! That's great!" I enthused.
"I'm not a rehab therapist, but I've seen lots of people go home right after they start practicing on the stairs."

"It couldn't happen soon enough for me!" Miguel replied. He smoothed his hair back down again. "I'm ready."

The Rehabilitation Connection

The main reason short-term residents are in the nursing home is to get in the best physical condition possible before going home. If you're making progress, occupational and physical therapies will continue, and you're not likely to be discharged until they're over. Hang in there! **It's far better to stay in the nursing home a little longer than you'd hoped and to be able to manage successfully in the community**, than it is to leave too soon, have trouble at home, and need to come back.

The following week, Miguel was triumphant. "Look at this!" He handed me an award certificate that showed he'd successfully completed his rehabilitation.

"Congratulations! Well done!" I told him. "I guess you'll be leaving us soon then."

"They're having a meeting with my cousin on Friday. I'm going home some time next week." He laced his hands together and held them behind his head. "I tell you, I didn't think this day would ever come!"

Discharge Planning Meeting

The team members, including your social worker, will meet with you and your family to discuss your needs in the community, such as a home health aide, visiting nurse, adaptive equipment, etc. The team will help you consider the realities of being at home and how to manage successfully.

For many people, the abilities they had before they came into the nursing home are not the abilities they have leaving the nursing home, no matter how successful the therapy. For example, a resident might have been able to walk independently prior to their health crisis and is being discharged with a cane or walker. One focus of the discharge-planning meeting will be on how such physical changes might affect life post-discharge.

Frequently, the trip to the nursing home has allowed some time and space for residents to reevaluate their home situation. **Perhaps they realize they were too isolated, for example, and might benefit from an adult day program** to add structure and assistance to their lives. The discharge-planning meeting is the place to address this, and your social worker will help set it up for you.

"Miguel," I said, "before you leave here, I want to talk to you a little more about your drinking. I know you spent a lot of time at the bar before your fall, and I wonder if you see a connection between your drinking and your fall."

Miguel didn't hesitate at all to reply.

"Yeah, I was drunk when I fell. No point in denying it."

I was surprised he was so forthcoming. He'd been more guarded when I'd broached the subject before. "So now that you'll be heading back home, are you planning to spend much time at the bar or are you looking to make a change?"

"You mean, quit drinking? I've been thinking about it," he admitted. "But I've tried so many times before." His fingers tousled his hair.

"But you haven't tried AA before," I pointed out. "Would it be okay if I gave you some information about Alcoholics Anonymous meetings in your area? They even have them in Spanish, if you'd feel more comfortable."

"Yeah, that would be okay. Thanks," he said, looking me square in the face. "I'll try AA this time. I don't want to fall and come back here again!"

"Yes, Miguel. Don't take this the wrong way," I smiled at him, "but I hope

not to see you again."

He laughed. "Yeah, I hope I don't see you again either."

Home Health Services

Many residents will require some assistance with basic care once they return home and will receive home visits offered by a nursing service. A nurse will evaluate you while you're in the nursing home to see how many hours and what type of care you'll need at home. People commonly have home health aides for several hours each day to help with bathing, dressing, meals, and other "activities of daily living." The home health service may also provide a nurse to monitor care on a regular basis. Depending on your needs and the visiting nurse program, additional rehabilitation and other services might be offered.

Take some time to find out what services will be offered and to think about what it will be like to have new people in your home. For instance, an aide can allow you the opportunity to return home, but having an aide with you at home will also be a big change in your environment. Some people will welcome the company and assistance, while others will need time to adjust to sharing their space.

Safe Discharges

The nursing home is legally responsible for making sure you'll be safe in your home. The good news is that everything will be set up for you in order to make sure your discharge is as successful as possible.

If the nursing home doesn't think your discharge is safe, however, it can't discharge you home. This could happen, for instance, when a resident needs two people to get in and out of bed, and there is no one at home to assist the home health aide with the transfers. In another example, the home health program won't take on a case if there is no family member or friend available as a back-up in the event of emergency. Another problematic situation is when the resident is unable to get up and down the stairs at home, posing a hazard in the event of a fire.

One of the most challenging situations is when a resident wants to return home, but circumstances make this difficult or impossible. Talk to your social worker and family members about the options available for you. Sometimes a person decides to move to senior housing or an assisted-living community or someone might decide to live with a family member or stay in the nursing home. By talking with your support system, you'll be able to find the best alternative for you.

Glossary

Activity Department—The activity department, also referred to as the recreation department, provides daily entertainment for you and will assist you in adapting activities to your ability level.

Activities of Daily Living (ADLs)—ADLs refer to tasks such as bathing, tooth brushing, getting dressed, toileting, and other hygiene-related tasks.

Administrator—The nursing home administrator is similar to a president. The administrator is in charge of running the facility on a day-to-day basis.

Certified Nursing Assistant (CNA)—The CNA assists you with ADLs (activities of daily living), such as getting you ready for the day and helping you to bed at night.

Charge Nurse—The charge nurse is "in charge" of the floor or unit, making sure residents get the care that's needed.

Dietitian—The dietician makes sure you have the types of foods you enjoy within the diet that is healthy for you.

Director of Nursing (DON)—The DON is in charge of all the nurses, nursing supervisors, and nursing assistants.

Medication Nurse—The medication nurse gives the medications to residents.

Nursing Supervisor—The nursing supervisor is generally in charge of the flow of nursing care for several floors or units, and supervises the charge nurses, medication nurses, and aides.

Occupational Therapy (OT)—The occupational therapist is part of the rehabilitation department, focusing on restoring skills and teaching how to use adaptive equipment so that residents can participate in everyday activities.

Physiatrist—A physiatrist is a physician that specializes in restoring optimal functioning to people with injuries or illness.

Physical Therapy (PT)—The physical therapist is part of the rehabilitation department and focuses on restoring your strength and fitness level, for instance, helping residents to walk again.

Psychiatrist—The psychiatrist is a physician who specializes in mental health disorders, often prescribing medication to improve or restore mental health functioning.

Psychologist—The psychologist is a doctoral-level mental health professional who talks to residents to assist them in coping with various aspects of nursing home life.

Recreation Department—The recreation department, also referred to as the activities department, provides daily entertainment for you and will assist you in adapting activities to your ability level.

Rehabilitation—Rehabilitation is the umbrella term for the services provided by the occupational and physical therapists.

Social Worker—The social worker is a mental health professional that works with you and your family on admission and discharge issues and any number of interpersonal and sometimes financial concerns that arise during your stay.

Speech Therapist—The speech therapist works with residents to restore functioning if speech is impaired and conducts swallowing evaluations to be sure you can eat safely.

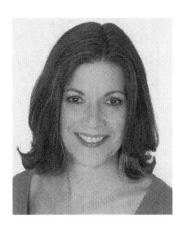

About Dr. El

Eleanor Feldman Barbera, PhD is an author, speaker, and consultant who has been sharing insights gleaned over fifteen years as a nursing home psychologist. She's been in resident rooms and at the nursing stations, talking with residents, families, line staff and administrators. She's spoken with policy makers and CEOs of large chain nursing homes, with researchers and watchdog agencies. She is a regular contributor to *Long-Term Living Magazine* and *McKnight's Long Term Care News*. Dr. El can teach you how to create a nursing home where EVERYBODY thrives.

Visit Dr. El at
MyBetterNursingHome.com